100 Simple
AFRICAN
Dishes

Discover Authentic Family Recipes from all over the Continent

Catherine Smith

DISCLAIMER

The recipes and nutritional advice provided in this book are for general informational purposes only. If you have special dietary needs or health concerns, please consult your dietitian or physician.

Please understand that this document is not intended to substitute for advice from a qualified medical professional. Please consult your physician or health care professional regarding any suggestions or recommendations contained in this document. By using this book, you agree to this disclaimer.

Allergen information and nutritional values listed here are approximate and may vary depending on the ingredients used. Readers with dietary restrictions are encouraged to have the information verified by an appropriate professional.

© 2024 Catherine Smith. All rights reserved.

TABLE OF CONTENTS

1. WEST AFRICAN FUFU 7
2. SUKUMA WIKI 10
3. IRIO 12
4. IRIO (RECIPE 2) 13
5. UGALI: 14
6. UGALI (CORNMEAL PORRIDGE) SECOND RECIPE 15
7. SERVINGS OF BEEF OR CHICKEN STEW 16
8. GITHERI - PRINCIPAL DISH 16
9. SUKUMA WIKI 18
10. PLANTAINS IN COCONUT MILK 20
11. KUNDE 21
12. KENYAN VERMICELLI BREAD 23
13. MATAHA (DRY MAIZE, BEANS AND POTATOES) 24
14. KENYAN CABBAGE 24
15. CHAPATIS 25
16. SWEETS MANDAZI 26
17. MAANDAZI (SWEET DOUGHNUT) RECIPE 2 27
18. COCONUT AND YAM PUDDING 28
19. SWEET RICE 29
20. HOT BANANA BREAD 30
21. BANANA PUDDING 31
22. ROADSTER MOUNT KENYA 32
23. PINEAPPLE RUM SAUCE 33
24. CRUNCHY N'DIZI (BANANAS) 33
25. CHILLED BANANA CREAM: (EGG CUSTARD) 34
26. CHAI (KENYAN TEA) 36

27.	"KARRINGMELK BESKUIT" RECIPE	36
28.	CAPE LIQUOR PUDDING RECIPE	37
29.	"KOEKSISTERS"	39
30.	MEALIE BREAD	40
31.	MILK TART	41
32.	"MOSBOLLETJIE"	43
33.	ROOSTERKOEK	44
34.	"SKILPADJIES"	46
35.	POTJIE	47
36.	HAMBURGER CURRY SOUP	48
37.	BILTONG &PEPPADEW TERRINE	49
38.	BILTONG	50
39.	BILTONG PASTA POTJIE RECIPE	54
40.	BILTONG POTJIE RECIPE	55
41.	BILTONG RECIPE	56
42.	BOBOTIE	57
43.	BOEREWORS (HISTORY)	59
44.	DROE "WORS" (DRIED WIENER) RECIPE	61
45.	DRY OXTAIL PIECES WITH PAPER TOWEL	64
46.	CHICKEN RABBIT CHOW	67
47.	CHICKEN CURRY POTJIE RECIPE	69
48.	CHICKEN PIE	70
49.	"MIELIE MEAL"	72
50.	FAST AND SIMPLE "MELKKOS" RECIPE	75
51.	SOUSKLUITJIES (DATED DUMPLINGS WITH CINNAMON AND SUGAR)	76
52.	FISH CAKES	77
53.	SNOEK WITH APRICOT JAM	78
54.	CURRIED FISH (SALTED FISH)	79

55.	DURBAN RABBIT CHOW	81
56.	GENTLE SHEEP CURRY POTJIE RECIPE	82
57.	SHEEP NECK AND CABBAGE "POTJIE"	83
58.	'KORINGSLAAI' (WHEAT) SALAD RECIPE	86
59.	CARROT "BREDIE" (STEW)	87
60.	CHAKALAKA	88
61.	COPPER PENNY CARROT SALAD RECIPE	90
62.	DICE GREEN PEPPERS OR CHILIES.	90
63.	CRUSHED DRY MAIZE/CORN KERNELS	91
64.	HONEY SIMMERED YAMS	92
65.	POUNDED BEANS RECIPE	93
66.	OLD FASHIONED BEAN SOUP	95
67.	SIAPHAKSKEENTJIES - TRADITIONAI SOUTH AFRICAN	96
68.	RECIPE FOR EAST AFRICAN PILAU AND KACHUMBARI	97
69.	KAIMATI (BROILED DUMPLINGS)	98
70.	MEAT SAMOSA (SAMBUSA YA NYAMA)	99
71.	WEST AFRICA JOLLOF RICE	101
72.	PILAU RICE	102
73.	CURRY POTATOES	104
74.	PUERTO RICO	106
75.	ATAKILT WAT ETHIOPIA	108
76.	LENTIL SAMBUSA ETHIOPIA	109
77.	MOIN MOI/MOI NIGERIA	111
78.	LENTIL SALAD MOROCCO	113
79.	MAFÉ SENEGAL	114
80.	CURRY GOAT JAMAICA	115
81.	WAAKYE GHANA	117
82.	SUYA	119

83.	PERI (OR PIRI) SOUTH AFRICA	120
84.	MOROCCO BRAISED SHEEP KNIFE	123
85.	KEY WATT HAMBURGER STEW ETHIOPIA	124
86.	JAMAICA JERK CHICKEN	127
87.	CHERMOULA FISH MOROCCO	129
88.	JAMAICA RUM CAKE	131
89.	KELEWELE	132
90.	PUFF-PUFF NIGERIA	133
91.	DUMPLINGS JAMAICA	135
92.	MANDAZI TANZANIA	137
93.	DAWADAWA JOLLOF WITH GUINEA FOWL	137
95.	TZ (TUO ZAAFI)	139
96.	WAAKYE (RICE AND BEANS)	140
97.	BUBBLED PIGEON PEA	141
98.	GROUNDNUT SOUP AT HOME MAIN DISHES (SOUPS AND STEWS)	142
99.	FISH BRA LEAVES SOUP	143
101.	COMMON NAMES FOR ADANSONIA DIGITATA:	148
102.	PRESENT WITH BANKU, EBA, KENKEY	149
103.	AMARANTH LEAVES STEW	151
104.	SABDARIFFA HIBISCUS	152
105.	SIMMERED GROUNDNUTS	153
106.	KOOSE (SEARED COWPEA BEAN CAKE)	155
107.	CORN MIXTURE FLOUR PORRIDGE	156
109.	FLAVORED SORGHUM BATTER PORRIDGE	157
110.	FLAVORED MILLET FLOUR PORRIDGE	157

100 SIMPLE AFRICAN DISHES

Numerous recipes are known in Africa and are passed down from generation to generation. The diversity of African recipes derives from the continent's cultural diversity, as each tribe has its own culinary traditions and traditions.

African cuisine is very diverse, with regional differences in the preparation and use of flavors, spices, and cooking procedures. This collection of African recipes introduces the rich food culture of the African people. Here are some of the most common African dishes you must try.

African food is very diverse and includes many different cultures from north to south and east to west. But no matter where you are on the continent, you can always find something delicious to eat.

To help you create these great flavors in your own kitchen, we've compiled a list of African recipes from Gypsy Plate and the internet.

Find everything here, from hearty soups and stews to fried and grilled meats, rice preparations, vegetable dishes and more.

Try making all these amazing African dishes...you'll adore the taste!

MUST-TRY AFRICAN DISHES:
1. WEST AFRICAN FUFU

Fufu is a totally well-known African dish that originated in West Africa, specifically Nigeria and Ghana. Follow these step-by-step instructions and you'll be able to make delicious fufu in your home kitchen, just like in your homeland.

Fufu – A simple, filling and hearty side dish that is easy to prepare. A perfect combination with soups/stews and proteins.

Ingredients

- Yuca root cassava 1 piece
- Plantain green 1 piece
- 1/4 cup water

How to make dough

Peel the cassava, cut the tuber in half lengthwise, and remove the inner woody core. , cut the potatoes into small cubes.

Peel the plantains and cut them into small cubes.

Place everything in a blender and blend until a smooth dough forms.

Stovetop Method

Pour the batter into a saucepan, place over medium heat, and begin stirring until a thick, pastry dough-like fufu forms.

Add water, cover and simmer over low to medium heat for 5 minutes. If you feel that the wheat gluten is not cooked through yet, please simmer it a little more. Mix well.

Divide the wheat gluten into different sizes and wrap in plastic wrap.

Enjoy with your favorite soup or stew.

Microwave method

Place the dough in a microwave-safe bowl and cover with a microwave-safe lid. Place in the microwave for 5 minutes.

Stir well until a smooth mixture forms.

Add some water and microwave again until done, about 5-8 minutes.

Stir again, divide into individual sized portions and wrap in plastic wrap.

Enjoy with your favorite soup or stew.

Notes

Please note that the fufu will harden as it cools. Therefore, it is better to cook it softer, especially if you are not going to eat it right away.

Nutrition

Calories: 218kcal

Carbohydrates: 53g

Protein: 2g

Fat: 1g

Saturated Fat: 1g

Sodium: 17 mg

Potassium: 500 mg

Dietary Fiber: 3g

Sugar: 8g

Vitamin A: 518 IU

Vitamin C: 29mg

Calcium: 18 mg

Iron: 1mg

2. SUKUMA WIKI

Perfect for a nice lunch or leisurely dinner, delicious, quick and healthy! It uses fewer ingredients, requires less effort, takes less time to cook, and produces delicious results. This is how to introduce kale and kale.

Sukuma Wiki

Sukuma Wiki is a nutritious and delicious vegetable dish that can be combined with a variety of meals.

This is one of the staple foods of Tanzanians and Kenyans. It's basically a vegetable stew, made with kale or collards, onions, tomatoes, and spices.

Sukuma Wiki is an inexpensive meal that is used in East Africa to extend meals to last a week, hence the name ``Sukuma Wiki," meaning ``to get through the week." I did.

Traditionally it is eaten with ugali/sazza, fried meat or fish, but I also like it with rice.

Ingredients for making oil – use those with a neutral flavor and high smoke point.

Chopped tomatoes - I like to use fresh, but canned tomatoes are also fine.

Kale or Kale - I always use fresh. You can use frozen ones, but fresh ones taste much better.

Salt and Bouillon Cubes – Flavor!!

Onions – Essential!!

Garlic – Optional

Beef – Optional

Chili Peppers – Adjust Spiciness – Totally Optional

How to Make Sukuma Wiki

To prepare kale, wash it. Pat dry, cut off thick stems, remove ribs and chop. Cut the sheet to the desired dimension.

Like most seasonings, Sukuma Wiki starts with finely chopped onions sautéed with salt and black pepper.

Brown and cook meat. If you are a vegetarian, you can omit the meat completely. Don't worry; your taste will still be delicious!

If you want to dry out the mixture before adding the kale or kale, stir-fry the diced tomatoes or paste.

Once you've added the kale or kale, you can cook it to your desired level of crispiness or tenderness, as desired.

Sukuma Wiki – A perfect dish for a nice lunch or leisurely dinner. Delicious, quick and healthy! It uses fewer ingredients, requires less effort, takes less time to prepare, and produces delicious results. This is how to introduce kale and kale.

Ingredients

- Oil tablespoons 2
- Chopped onion
- beef 1.5 pound
- Medium tomato 2 pieces
- Salt
- beef buin cube or 1 chicken
- chicken kale or kale 8 cups

How to make Fries

Heat the oil Sauté the additional onions until golden brown, about 5 minutes.

Supplement the red meat and season with salt and bouillon cube. Stir often and cook until tender.

Add tomatoes and cook until tomatoes are soft, about 3 minutes.

Add the kale or kale and cook until the leaves are soft.

3. IRIO

Fundamentally a combination of pureed potatoes, peas and corn (maize), it is a conventional dish among the Kikuyu nation of Kenya. In fact, the word for food in Kikuyu is the name of this dish. Generally filled in as a side dish to a meat dish

Servings: 8-10

Planning Time: 30 minutes

Ingredients

- 1 onion
- 5 lb (2.5 kg) of potatoes stripped and cleaved minuscule
- 1 lb (500g) of green peas (can utilize tinned handled peas - use tins to make up approx. weight.

Cooking Instructions: Drain well 1/2 lb (250 g) of sweet corn or the closest size tin. Add spices and vegetable oil.

1. Sear the finely hacked onion in a little vegetable oil to a light brilliant variety in a pot.

2. Add the stripped potatoes to the pot and cover with bubbling water.

3. Add sweet corn, peas, and salt if desired when almost cooked. Let bubble for 2 to 5 minutes

4. Crush the combination until potatoes are smooth. It ought to look a wonderful pea-green variety.

4. IRIO (RECIPE 2)

Ingredients

- 1 teacup dehydrated peas (or canned peas)
- 1 lb canned corn or 6 ears of new corn
- A few potatoes or moment pureed potatoes
- ½ lb pumpkin greens or spinach
- Lima Beans (discretionary)
- Hacked broiled onions (discretionary)
- Dark pepper
- Salt

Bubble dried peas until détente, channel and put away. Additionally heat up the potatoes, corn, lima beans, and the greens, channel and put away.

Blend the seared onions in with all the above mentioned, add salt and pepper to taste and squash.

The consistency should be that of mashed potatoes. If you like, you can also add a little bit of butter.

The extras taste extraordinary the following day when seared with a touch of oil in a container.

5. UGALI:

Ugali is to Kenyan cooking what squashed potato is to the English aside from all the more broadly eaten - for example with most dinners. Ugali is like Southern Africa's Mealie-feast, Nshima, and Sadza.

In West Africa it is called Fufu.

It is typically produced using maize (corn) which was brought from the Americas to Africa by Europeans. Millet was used to make it in the past. It is a dull backup for the African soup or stew or sauce, or different dishes with sauce or sauce. Ugali is by and large made by bubbling furthermore; overwhelmingly mixing a boring fixing into a thick, smooth mush. Numerous Kenyans feel they haven't had a feast except if they have eaten Ugali with a sauce or stew.

Ingredients

- 6 cups of water.
- 4 cup of maize flour or white cornmeal that has been finely ground - accessible in ethnic basic food item shops - (You can likewise substitute semolina)

Headings:

Heat water to bubbling in a pot, slowly empty ½ the corn flour into bubbling water mixing consistently to keep away from bumps.

Mix constantly and pound any bumps that truly do frame until bubbling.

Permit to bubble for around 10 minutes mixing periodically.

Presently for the difficult work: Add more corn flour bit by bit, blending constantly until it is thicker and drier than pureed potatoes - it ought to pull away from the sides of the dish.

Cook for three or four minutes, keeps on mixing. (Proceeding to mix as the ugali thickens is the little-known technique, i.e., bump free ugali.)

Tip the ugali into a bowl that has been wetted before serving. For a truly real see, quickly tenderly 'flip' the ugali so the base side is currently up and it looks smooth.

Cover and keep warm.

Serve promptly with any meat, or vegetable stew, or any dish with a sauce or sauce. It is frequently eaten with your right hand - sever a piece, fold it into a ball, make a space what's more, gather up the stew or sauce.

6. UGALI (CORNMEAL PORRIDGE) SECOND RECIPE

The ugali will be done when it pulls from the sides of the dish effectively and doesn't stick. It ought to seem to be solid corn meal.

Ingredients

- 1 cup cold water
- 1 cup yellow cornmeal (the Mexican flour 'Mozerapa' is a nearby substitute to the Kenyan flour) - or substitute semolina
- 1 teaspoon salt (discretionary)
- 3 cups bubbling water

Put cold water in a medium-size pot; add cornmeal and salt, blending persistently. Bring to a bubble over high intensity, continuously blending and gradually add 3 cups of bubbling water to forestall protuberances.

Cover and cook for about 8 minutes at a simmer, stirring frequently to prevent sticking.

You can serve ugali including meat stew to sugar and cream. Your decision!

7. SERVINGS OF BEEF OR CHICKEN STEW

Planning Time: 60 minutes

Ingredients

- 1 lb. meat cut into shapes or chicken pieces
- 2 carrots
- 2 green peppers
- 4 tomatoes/tinned tomatoes
- 2 onions hacked sprinkle Ground Coriander
- ½ tspn gentle Curry powder
- Dark pepper and salt
- Meat or chicken stock

Cooking Directions:

Fry the meat until it is brown and season to taste. Eliminate from the skillet.

The onions should be fried until soft. Include chopped green pepper and tomatoes. Add carrots, dark pepper, coriander and curry powder. At the point when the carrots have become somewhat delicate add the meat and stock. Curry powder and salt to taste should be added to the meat when it is almost done.

On the other hand, when every one of the vegetables and meat has been broiled, you could move it to a goulash dish and cook in the broiler. Hamburger especially will profit from a low, slow cooking.

8. GITHERI - PRINCIPAL DISH

Githeri is essential maize (corn) and beans stew, customary among the Kikuyu nation of Kenya.

In addition to the fact that these two eaten together are, they are frequently intercropped (become together) in the same fields. At its least difficult, githeri is simply maize and beans. In some cases potatoes, greens (kale or on the other hand comparative), or meat are added.

Planning Time: 45 minutes Ingredients for the dish:

Dried entire part corn (maize); cold-water-rinsed dried beans (kidney beans or something similar); absorbed cold water for a couple of hours, flushed

Cooking Guidelines:

Combine equal amounts of dried corn and beans in a large pot. Add sufficient virus water to cover. Heat to the point of boiling and cook over high intensity for ten minutes.

Lessen heat. Cover and stew for two hours or until corn and beans are delicate. In the completed dish, the vast majority of the water ought to be retained, and the corn and beans ought to be delicate yet still flawless, not soft. Add salt, fat, or oil to taste.

Hot, serve as a side dish or as a main dish on its own.

Ingredients for Vegetable Curry:

- 2 large, finely chopped onions, 2 tablespoons oil
- 1 tsp. cumin seeds
- 1 tsp. mustard seeds, preferably of the black variety; eight medium potatoes, quartered; one and a half teaspoon fresh ginger, minced and crushed 1 large garlic clove, 1 tablespoon 1 tablespoon ground cumin crushed whole coriander, two chili peppers, or one teaspoon cayenne pepper
- 1/2 tsp. 1 teaspoon turmeric 4 cinnamon sticks, 6 cloves, and 4 oz. of salt tomato paste, 1 pound green beans

- 1/2 of a little cauliflower 1 medium eggplant
- 1/2 lb. shelled fresh green peas or one small package of frozen green peas, one bunch of fresh leafy greens (such as kale, spinach, or collards), or one small bag of frozen greens and one cup cooked dried chickpeas (optional). Preheat the oven to 350 degrees. In a huge, weighty skillet or pot, brown the onions in tolerably hot oil alongside the cumin seeds and mustard seeds.

Stir the spices into the potato pieces (peeling is optional) before adding them. Presently add the excess flavors and keep on mixing for a few minutes.

Dainty the tomato glue with around 2/3 cup of water, Mix into the pot, Add vegetables, one at a time, cooking briefly or so between every expansion, and set in the cooked chickpeas last.

Transfer the mixture to an oven-proof pot if yours is not.

Cover with a top or seal with foil and prepare for around 45 minutes, really taking a look at after the initial 20 minutes.

The consistency ought to be somewhat thick, yet add fluid if important to forestall consuming. Mix periodically to forestall staying.

Serve over rice or with Indian bread.

9. SUKUMA WIKI

The Swahili expression Sukuma Wiki implies push the week - - what's truly being pushed is the family food spending plan. This is an extraordinary method for spending extra meat by joining it with greens and a couple of different fixings to make an exquisite dish. In Africa this dish may be made with greens like kale or collards; however it can likewise be made with cassava leaves, yam leaves, or pumpkin leaves. It also tastes good without meat.

Ingredients

- 2lb/1kg of greens (kale, collards, spinach, or comparative), very much cleaned and cleaved in to enormous pieces; (frozen greens can be utilized if they are defrosted first)
- two tablespoons flour
- juice of one lemon
- oil for searing
- one onion, cleaved
- a few tomatoes, cleaved (or canned entire tomatoes, depleted)
- one chile pepper, cleaved (discretionary)
- extra cooked meat: hamburger, chicken, or comparative (discretionary)
- salt, cayenne pepper or red pepper

What you do

Heat two cups of water to the point of boiling in an enormous pot. Place greens in a pot. Cover and steam until greens are almost delicate. While greens are cooking: consolidate flour, lemon juice, what's more, a couple of spoonful of water in a little bowl or cup. Mix vivaciously until blend is smooth. Eliminate greens from intensity and channel.

Heat oil in a different skillet

Sauté the onion, tomatoes, and hot pepper together. Add flavors to taste. Add meat. Add flour-lemon juice combination and mix until smooth.

Decrease heat. Add depleted greens. Cover and stew over low intensity until greens are completely delicate and sauce is thickened.

Great presented with Ugali

10. PLANTAINS IN COCONUT MILK

Ingredients

- 3-4 plantains, cut in adjusts
- ¼ teaspoon of salt
- 1 teaspoon of curry powder
- ½ teaspoon of cinnamon 1/8
- teaspoon cloves
- 1-2 cups of coconut milk

Join all fixings, with the exception of the coconut milk, in a weighty pan and mix. Pour in 1 cup of coconut milk and stew over low intensity until the plantains ingested the milk and are very delicate. A significant chunk of time must pass for them to get delicate; Give them roughly the same amount of time as you would for potatoes.

You can add more coconut milk assuming you want.

Serve hot and attempt with fish or curries.

Note: The brilliant thing about plantains is that they really are a flexible food. As a plantain ages, its high starch content changes to sugar.

Plantains are great at any stage; it simply relies upon what you need to make. Plantains are related to bananas, but because they are larger and less sweet, they must be cooked before eating.

In contrast to bananas, which become mushy when cooked, plantains retain their shape.

Green or "unripe" plantains contain a great deal of starch and very little pleasantness. Their boring tissue is involved more as a vegetable than an organic product. They can be boiled, mashed, or added to stews and soups.

Savory and sweet dishes can be made with a ripe plantain. You can sauté them with some spread, rum, and earthy colored sugar and serve over frozen yogurt. While purchasing ready plantains, they ought to be firm and not soft or broke.

While stripping plantains or green bananas, saturate hands and rub with salt to forestall the juices from adhering to your hands.

The plantain should have about an inch of cutoff at both ends.

Cut the plantain in half lengthwise in two places at opposite ends with a sharp knife.

While holding the plantain consistent with your left hand, utilize your right hand to slide the tip of the blade under the skin and start to pull it away, going through and through.

Absorb the stripped plantains or bananas salted water.

Channel on a paper towel to use in your recipe.

11. KUNDE

(Kenyan dark looked at peas and tomatoes)

Ingredients

- 2 teaspoons Oil
- 1 Onion
- 2 cups tomatoes

- 2 cups dark peered toward peas
- 1/4 cup peanut butter, normal or generally grounded peanuts ¼ cup water
- Salt and Pepper

Heat oil over medium intensity in a pan

Mince onions and sauté daintily until clear. Add diced tomatoes and stew around 5 minutes to cook down.

Cook the dark peered toward peas and ads with every excess fixing and blends well. With a fork, lightly mash the peas.

Stew around 10 minutes over medium intensity, blending at times. Add more water depending on the situation to get a stew-like consistency.

Serve alongside rice.

Ingredients for Kenyan-style mixed greens:

- 1 Serrano or Jalapeno pepper, hacked
- 2 teaspoons salt
- 2 teaspoons newly grounded dark pepper
- 2 tablespoons olive oil
- 1 pound new collard, mustard or turnip greens, hacked

Or on the other hand

- 1 sack/10 ounces frozen cleaved greens, defrosted
- 1 pound new spinach, hacked

Or on the other hand

- 1 sack/10 ounces frozen cleaved spinach, defrosted and pressed dry
- 2 tablespoons margarine

- 3 huge tomatoes, cubed
- 1 huge yellow onion, stripped and cleaved
- 1 cup canned unsweetened coconut milk
- 4 teaspoons dry broiled peanuts, cleaved (discretionary)

Fill a huge pot half-full with water. Salt, black pepper, and one tablespoon of the olive oil should be added. Heat to the point of boiling over high intensity. Add the greens and spinach. Decrease the intensity to low and cook for 20 minutes, mixing sporadically.

In a large skillet, melt the butter and the remaining 1 tablespoon of oil over medium heat. Simmer the milk, greens and spinach, tomatoes, and onions for ten minutes, stirring occasionally. Taste the greens for delicacy and preparing. Cook for 10 extra minutes and add seriously preparing, if necessary. If desired, sprinkle with the peanuts.

12. KENYAN VERMICELLI BREAD

Ingredients

12 pound vermicelli (thin pasta) 4 cups unsweetened coconut milk 12 cup sugar 14 teaspoon ground ginger 1 egg 12 cup whole wheat or all-purpose flour Serves 12 Preheat the oven to 350 degrees Fahrenheit. Coat a baking dish that is 13 by 9 inches with butter or cooking spray.

Set up the vermicelli as indicated by the bundle heading and channel.

Heat the coconut milk and sugar in an enormous pot over medium intensity. Stir the mixture constantly as you bring it to a boil. Cook for five minutes at a low heat. Add the vermicelli also, ginger.

In a small bowl, beat the egg. Add 1 or 2 tablespoons of the coconut milk blend to the beaten egg, and afterward mix the egg blend into the skillet with the vermicelli. Speed in the flour what's more; empty the combination into the pre-arranged baking dish.

Bake for one hour, or until the sponge is soft. It can be cut into squares or any other shape that works for you.

13. MATAHA (DRY MAIZE, BEANS AND POTATOES)

Ingredients

- ½ pound dried red beans
- 1 pound dried maize (corn)
- Salt
- 8 medium potatoes, stripped and cubed
- 10 pumpkin leaves(or spinach), coarsely hacked

Splash the beans and maize short-term in water to cover. Add salt, cover with water once more, drain, and boil for 22 hours. Channel and put away. Cover the potatoes with water and bubble until delicate. Add the pumpkin leaves and cook until delicate. Drain. Add to the maize and beans and squash all together. The mixture ought to be firm and thick.

14. KENYAN CABBAGE

Ingredients

- 2 medium tomatoes, hacked
- ½ medium onion, hacked
- 2 tbsp vegetable oil

- 1 little green cabbage, hacked

Sear the tomatoes and onions in the oil until the onions are brown. Add the cabbage also, mix over low intensity. Cook for 2 to 3 seconds. The cabbage ought to be a piece fresh when served. Present with Rice, Ugali and meat of your decision.

You can substitute the cabbage with sukuma wiki or spinach

15. CHAPATIS

Chapatis are regularly used to go with stews and vegetables.

Ingredients

- 1 Cup white flour
- 1 Cup whole-wheat flour
- 1/2 teaspoon salt
- 1 Tablespoon oil
- water to make a mixture
- 1 Tablespoon mellowed margarine or ghee

Filter flours and salt together in bowl. Make stiff dough by combining enough cold water with oil. Ply for 5-8 minutes until smooth and flexible. Cover with a soggy fabric and let it stand 2-3 hours. Work once more and separation into balls, around 3-4 cm in width. Roll into level hotcakes with oil, margarine or ghee. Cook the chapati in the pan until it starts to puff up. Using a spatula, press the cake to help it puff up. This guarantees light and cushy chapatis. Turnover and do it all over again. Eliminate from the container and spot in foil or fabric, spreading margarine on top of every chapati. Serve right away.

16. SWEETS MANDAZI

Mandazi (or Maandazi, additionally called Mahamri or Mamri) are East African seared breads like doughnuts. They are eaten with tea or espresso for breakfast, as a tidbit, or with the principal course for lunch or supper. They are not as sweet as doughnuts and don't have a sugar coating or icing.

Planning Time: 1.5 hours

Ingredients for the recipe:

4 oz (115g) granulated sugar 1/4 tsp mixed spice (or any mix of cardamom, cinnamon, allspice, or ginger) 2 tbs butter, margarine, or vegetable oil 2 fl.oz (60ml) warm milk (optional) 1 egg, lightly beaten, pinch of salt Oil for deep frying Instructions for Cooking:

If the ingredients have been in the refrigerator, they should be allowed to come to room temperature. If yeast is used: blend the yeast in with a couple of spoonful of the warm water.

If you are not using yeast, combine the flour, baking powder, sugar, and spice in a bowl (cardamom is most common in Eastern Africa). Put the yeast in. Combine the milk, egg, butter (or margarine, or oil), and water. While kneading the mixture into dough, gradually add this mixture to the flour. On the off chance that not utilizing milk and egg utilize extra water as required.) Manipulate until a smooth and flexible batter is framed - - fifteen to twenty minutes. If yeast is used: Place batter in a spotless bowl, cover with a material, and permit to ascend in a warm spot for an hour or more. In the case of utilizing baking powder, let mixture rest for a few minutes.

Divide the dough into several pieces the size of a hand. Roll or press the pieces into circles around one-half inch thick. Cut circles into equal parts or quarters (or anything you like). A few cooks (while utilizing yeast) put the mixtures on a treat sheet and let them rise a subsequent time.

Heat vegetable oil to 150C in a profound pot or profound fat fryer. Sear the mixtures in the hot oil, turning a couple of times, until they are brilliant earthy colored everywhere. Fry only the ones that can float in the oil together without touching. Put on paper towels to deplete. Keep warm.

17. MAANDAZI (SWEET DOUGHNUT) RECIPE 2

Ingredients

- (Makes around 30 laptops)
- 1 cup spread (or margarine)
- 5 tbsp sugar
- 2 huge eggs, beaten
- ½ cup milk
- 6 ground cardamom seed
- 2 tsp baking powder
- 4 ½ cups generally useful wheat flour
- ½ cup water
- 6 cups vegetable oil

Combine and speed as one margarine and sugar. Mix in the milk and eggs. Add the cardamom and the baking powder. Combine the water and flour. Add extra flour if the dough is sticky. Manipulate well until batter is smooth and delicate. Cut the batter into 3 balls and carry out each to around 12 creeps in width and ¼ inch thick. Cut into squares and slice into 2-inch strips. Heat the oil in a profound skillet. To test if the oil is sufficiently hot, drop one mandaazi. In the event that it sinks, floats to the top, the oil is prepared.

In the pan, cook the mandarin one piece at a time without crowding them too much. Turn them frequently until they are brilliant brown. Drain the pan, and then cool.

Present with hot milk, espresso or tea (chai).

Six servings of tropical fruit dessert: one large pawpaw that has been peeled, seeded, and sliced; two large bananas that have been sliced; four passion fruits; juice from one lime or two lemons. Place the passion fruit in a large bowl. Add the pawpaw, and bananas. Throw together tenderly. Pour the lemon or lime and throw once more. Serve into little natural product bowls.

18. COCONUT AND YAM PUDDING

Ingredients

- 1 cup new ground coconut
- 1 ½ cups yams, bubbled or squashed
- 2 eggs
- ¾ cup sugar ¾
- cup milk ½
- cup water
- 4 tbsp softened spread
- ½ tsp blended flavors ½
- tsp cinnamon

Blend sugar, yams and coconut along with spoon until smooth. Add margarine, milk, water and beat completely. After lightly beating the eggs, gradually incorporate the mixture. Add cinnamon and spices. Keep beating until smooth and exceptionally smooth. Fill a greased baking dish with the mixture, and bake for 30 minutes in a hot oven until golden brown. It can be served cold or hot.

19. SWEET RICE

Ingredients

- cups rice
- 4½ cups water
- Touch of salt
- ¼ teaspoon orange food shading 4
- tbsp vegetable oil
- 8 cardamom units
- 1 ½ cups sugar
- ½ cup cut almonds
- ½ cup currants

Directions

Wash and flush the rice. Heat 4 cups water to the point of boiling and add the rice, salt and food shading, also, turn the intensity low. At the point when the water is half finished, channel off the water and put rice away. In a saucepan, heat the oil and combine the cardamom, sugar, and the remaining 12 cups of water. Bubble together until a thick syrup structures and add it to the rice in its skillet, mixing great to guarantee that the rice is well covered with syrup. Cover the rice and stew the rice an additional 10 minutes over low intensity, until the rice is still somewhat firm. Mix in the almonds and currants.

20. HOT BANANA BREAD

Ingredients

- 1 ½ cup Flour
- 1 cup granulated sugar
- ½ cup Spread or margarine
- 4 ready Bananas
- 2 Eggs
- 1 tsp Pop
- ½ tsp Salt
- ½ tsp Vanilla

Technique

Preheat broiler to 350F (180C)

Strip the bananas and squash well with a fork.

Add the eggs to the bowl and mix well.

Cream the spread, sugar and vanilla together in a blending bowl.

Crease in the beaten eggs and afterward the crushed bananas, it is well to guarantee that the combination consolidated.

Filter the dry fixings (flour, pop and salt) together and overlay into the creamed banana blend.

Delicately oil a portion tin and residue the lubed surface with flour.

Empty the banana bread blend into the portion tin and spot in the preheated stove.

Prepare for an hour

Permit to cool.

Take the banana bread out of the loaf tin and serve it sliced or buttered.

Can clearly be eaten cold, yet is totally delightful eaten somewhat warm

21. BANANA PUDDING

This banana pudding recipe is an alternative but interesting banana dessert. Which is light and simple to do?

Ingredients

- Ready bananas
- 2 eggs
- ½ cup granulated white sugar
- 1 tbsp lemon juice
- 1 pkt lemon, orange or apricot jam powder.
- Water as required

Technique

Strip and pound the bananas with a fork and quickly add the lemon juice

Separate the eggs

Heat up the amount of water determined in the guidelines on the jam parcel

Set up the jam as indicated by these guidelines.

Whisk the egg yolks with the sugar until foamy. Slowly add the egg/sugar mixture to the jelly mixture that is heating in a double boiler over boiling water. Add the bananas to the jelly mixture. Mix constantly while adding the combination.

Keep warming until the egg sugar combination disintegrates totally in the jam blend

Eliminate the jam combination from the intensity and cool

In the meantime beat the egg whites until they structure firm pinnacles

At the point when the banana jams combination starts to set overlap in the beaten egg whites

Fill a form and chill until set.

This banana pudding is flavorful with lashings of whipped cream

22. ROADSTER MOUNT KENYA

(Mango Frozen yogurt with punch!)

Ingredients:

4 to 5 ripe mangoes 1 cup heavy cream, 2 cups sugar, 2 tablespoons lemon peel, cut into small ribbons, 2 cups condensed milk, and 2 teaspoons salt. Peel, pit, and mash the mangoes. You ought to wind up with around 2 cups.

Whip the weighty cream with the sugar until firm.

In a 2-quart bowl join the 2 cups of squashed mangos, the lemon strip strips, dense milk and salt. Crease in the whipped cream.

Fill cooler plate or a 6-cup shape and freeze.

23. PINEAPPLE RUM SAUCE

Ingredients:

- 1 cup pineapple juice, canned
- 1 cup sugar
- ½ cup cooled white rum
- 3 cups new pineapple cut in ½ inch dices
- 1 tablespoon pistachio nuts

In a 1-quart sauce container stew the pineapple juice and the sugar, until it breaks down and structures into syrup.

Add the white rum and cool.

Pour the pineapple rum sauce over the cut fresh pineapple pieces in a 2-quart bowl. Marinate for a few hours.

Place 1 scoop Mango Frozen yogurt in a 6 oz wine glass. Top with 3 to 4 oz of Pineapple Rum Combination.

Embellish with pistachio nuts, coarsely hacked.

The rest is history!

Note: For the Coupe Mount Kenya, any fruit ice cream will do especially peach ice cream.

Additionally, fruit sherbet can be used. Canned pineapple might be filling in for the new, yet it is simply not calm something similar.

24. CRUNCHY N'DIZI (BANANAS)

Ingredients

- 8 Bananas, stripped
- 125 g/4 oz margarine, softened
- 125 g/4 oz groundnuts/peanuts, slashed

Steam the bananas in an enormous pan until warmed through; that will just require a couple of moments.

Be cautious that they don't turn out to be excessively delicate.

After draining, roll each one separately in the chopped groundnuts or peanuts before rolling in the melted butter.

Organize them on a baking dish and prepare in the broiler for 15 minutes at 190C/375F.

This works perfectly with frozen yogurt, particularly the Mango frozen yogurt referenced before!!

25. CHILLED BANANA CREAM: (EGG CUSTARD)

Ingredients

- 250 ml/8 oz milk
- 2 eggs
- 30 g/2 tbl spoons caster sugar
- 2 - 3 drops vanilla quintessence

Heat the milk nearly to the limit; however don't really allow it to bubble. Blend or whisk the eggs into the hot milk, then add the sugar and vanilla extract to make a smooth mixture. Stew gradually on extremely low intensity, mixing constantly until it thickens into smooth custard. Eliminate from the intensity and set to the side.

Ingredients: (Banana Cream) Egg Custard 2 very ripe bananas, thoroughly mashed 15 g/1 tbsp sugar (optional) 250 ml/8 oz whipped cream 3 to 4 drops food coloring (optional) Combine the egg custard, mashed bananas, and additional sugar. Mix in the whipped cream and the food shading. Move into a serving dish and freeze. Serve decorated with a fresh banana cut into attractive shapes. – Four Brandy Snaps per serving Ingredients:

- 4 oz Spread
- ½ cup sugar
- ½ cup corn syrup
- ½ tablespoon ground ginger
- 1/3 cup regular flour
- 3 tablespoons cognac
- 1 16 ounces whipped cream
- Makes 25 cognac snaps

Join the margarine, sugar, corn syrup and ground ginger in a container and mix over heat until well blended. Cool for 10 minutes.

Add the flour and mix into blend. Empty blend by spoonfuls into level lubed container, 3 to 4 inches separated.

Prepare at 350F until snaps straighten. Eliminate cautiously with spatula and, when marginally cooled, roll up into a cylinder.

Join the liquor with the whipped cream. Stuff tubes with liquor blend utilizing a cake pack.

Note: Liquor Snaps were initially presented by the English and they are without a doubt hair-raising treats. Be careful, you might become addicted to those!

26. CHAI (KENYAN TEA)

Drinks Ingredients for Chai (Kenyan Tea) 1 cup water 12 teaspoons of tea leaves (or one tea bag) 1 cup milk 2 to 4 teaspoons of sugar Heat the water and tea leaves together in a saucepan that is 3 to 4 quarts in size until they come to a boil.

Mix in the milk and sugar and cook until the limit of the milk. Eliminate and strain the Chai into a tea container or pot. Present with bread, mandazi or chapati.

BUTTERMILK RUSKS
27. "Karringmelk Beskuit" recipe

This is a customary rusk - extraordinary for dunking in your tea or espresso promptly in the first part of the day when you watch the sun ascend as the "Boer adventurers or Voortrekkers" did each day when they headed out from the Cape to the Transvaal.

In the event that the rusks are to be saved for quite a while, don't substitute margarine for the spread.

In the event that no buttermilk or yogurt is accessible, utilize new milk soured with lemon squeeze or white vinegar.

Ingredients

- 375g margarine
- 500g sugar
- An additional 2 enormous eggs
- 1,5kg self-rising flour
- 30ml (2 tablespoons) baking powder

- 500ml (2 cups) buttermilk or simple consuming yogurt
- Preheat broiler to 180°C.

Cream the margarine and sugar together well indeed. Add the eggs, each in turn. Using a fork, combine the flour and baking powder that have been sifted together with the creamed mixture. Add the buttermilk or yogurt, utilizing a little milk to wash out the container. Blend well in with a fork and afterward manipulate delicately. Bake for 45 to 55 minutes, close together, lightly rolled golf ball-sized buns from the dough in the greased bread pans. Place the dish in the broiler, with a sheet of earthy colored paper on the first rate to shield the buns from becoming caramelized excessively fast.

After the buns have cooked all the way through and are well risen, remove the paper to brown the tops.

Decrease the intensity to the least conceivable setting. Turn out the buns on to cake racks, cool them also, and separate them, utilizing 2 forks. Pack them on wire racks or on cooled broiler racks - air must circle. Place them in the cool broiler, leaving the entryway partially open, for 4-5 hours, or short-term, to dry out.

28. CAPE LIQUOR PUDDING RECIPE

Ideal for a change from the customary Christmas pud, this one has a South African bend and can be presented with cream or custard!

Ingredients

- 250g dates, generally cleaved
- 250 ml water
- 5ml bicarbonate of pop
- 100g spread, mellowed

- 200ml caster sugar
- 1 egg
- 250ml plain flour
- 5ml baking powder
- 100g walnut nuts, cleaved
- For the syrup:
- 250ml sugar
- 120ml water
- 120ml cognac
- 5ml vanilla pith
- 30ml spread
- 1/2 tsp ground cinnamon

Strategy

Preheat the stove to 180C and oil a broiler resistant dish.

Consolidate the dates with the water in a little pot and bring to the bubble. Add the bicarbonate of soda after taking the mixture off the heat.

Beat the egg, sugar, and butter together. Filter the flour and baking powder and add to the creamed combine as one with the cooled dates and blend well.

Blend in the nuts and fill the lubed dish. Heat for about an hour or until a stick comes out clean

For the syrup, heat up the sugar, water, margarine and vanilla quintessence together for around 10 minutes.

Add the cognac and cinnamon and blend well.

Serve the pudding with the syrup poured over it and top with some whipped cream (or on the other hand custard whenever liked).

29. "KOEKSISTERS"

Ingredients

- 250 ml (1 cup) cake flour
- 250 ml (1 cup) self-rising flour
- 5 ml (1 tsp.) salt
- 60g (1/4 cup) margarine
- 5 ml (1tsp) ground ginger
- 5 ml (1 tsp.) ground cinnamon
- 5 ml (1 tsp.) ground blended flavor
- 2.5 ml (1/2 tsp.) 10 ml (2 tsp.) ground cardamom delicate earthy colored sugar
- 10 ml (2 tsp.) white sugar
- 7.5 ml (1 1/2 tsp.) moment dry yeast
- 375 ml (1 1/2 cup) hot water

Syrup

Make syrup the other day and refrigerate. While broiling ttketkikterk", tate kut kf cooler and place in a compartment which is layered with ice solid shapes at the base.

- 250ml (1 cup) water
- 125ml (1/2 cup) sugar
- 15ml (1 tbsp.) parched coconut
- 1 piece of "naartjie" strip

To make the syrup bring, water, sugar, coconut and "naartjie" strip to a sluggish bubble in an enormous pan until syrup begins to bubble.

Strategy Batter

In a blending bowl consolidate the flours with salt.

Add spread and focus on delicately till it looks like fine breadcrumbs. Add remaining fixings, utilizing the warm water to shape mixture.

Try not to work. Cover with plastic and leave in a warm spot for around 1/1/2 to 2 hours or rose until multiplied in size then, at that point, turn out on a softly floured surface.

Dunk fingers and blade into flour and utilize your hands to extend the mixture.

Cut into 4 cm x 8 cm strips and deep fry in a large saucepan over medium heat.

Embed fork to check whenever done, and eliminate rapidly individually and channel in colander or on kitchen paper.

Prick each "koeksister", and afterward lower into syrup. As many "koeksisters" as the pan can accommodate, add. Turn and cook for 5 minutes each side or till sautéed. Eliminate with opened spoon place on platter with some additional coconut. Sprinkle coconut on top and serve warm.

30. MEALIE BREAD

Ingredients

1 1/2 cups thawed frozen corn kernels, 2 eggs, and 2 tablespoons melted butter 1 cup flour 2 teaspoons baking powder

2 Tbsp. 1/2 teaspoon sugar salt

Readiness:

Preheat stove to 350°F and grease portion pans.

Mix 1 cup of corn, the eggs, and dissolved margarine together until a coarse blend structures.

Add the leftover 1/2 cup of corn and heartbeat the blend a couple of additional times.

Leave numerous parts entirety.

Mix flour, baking powder, sugar and salt.

Utilizing a huge spoon, join the dry fixings with corn combination until a thick blend structures.

Add it to your portion dish and prepare around 30 to 35 minutes.

Permit the bread to cool somewhat prior to cutting.

31. MILK TART

A custom made South African "melktert" is generally a champ. Whether you really want dessert for your evening gathering, a cake for a unique event or essentially a cut of something sweet with your midday cup of tea - this simple "melktert" recipe will figure you out.

Ingredients - baked well:

- 2 cups flour
- 1 egg
- 1/2 cup sugar
- 2 tsp baking powder
- 125g spread touch of salt

Strategy - cake:

Add the egg after thoroughly combining the butter and sugar.

Add any remaining fixings - making solid mixture.

Press into a couple of round cake tins/pie dishes and prepare at 180°C until light brown.

Ingredients - filling:

- 1/2 cups milk
- ½ tbsp. corn flour
- 1 cup sugar
- 3 eggs touch of salt
- ½ tbsp flour
- 1 tsp vanilla embodiment a major spoon of spread

Strategy - filling:

- Carry milk to the bubble.
- Beat eggs well, add sugar, flour, cornmeal, and salt and mix.
- Blend well.
- Add boiling milk to the mixture and thoroughly stir. Get back to oven and mix well until blend thickens.

Add spread and vanilla substance and fill cooked shell.

Permit to cool in the refrigerator (you don't have to cook the tart any further) to adorn, sprinkle with cinnamon.

32. "MOSBOLLETJIE"

The most ideal way to portray "mosbolletjies" is that it's a sweet brioche, customarily made with aged grape squeeze (nowadays we simply utilize typical grape squeeze) and seasoned with aniseed.

There's nothing quite like a torn piece of mosboregge, which has a cushioned surface and is coated thickly with margarine and glossy syrup.

Ingredients

- 1 kg cake flour
- 10 ml salt
- 100 g sugar
- 10 g moment dry yeast
- 30 ml entire aniseed
- 250 ml white grape juice
- 125 ml tepid milk
- 250 ml tepid water
- 30 ml sugar blended in with 30 ml tepid water (sugar syrup for brushing in the wake of baking)

Technique

Filter flour and salt together. Add sugar, yeast and aniseed. Mix well.

In a saucepan, heat the grape juice and butter until the butter is melted. Try not to bubble. Add to dry fixings alongside milk and water, and then blend to shape a delicate mixture.

Turn out batter on a daintily floured surface, then manipulate for 5-10 minutes, or until the mixture is delicate and versatile. Place in a huge oiled bowl, then, at that point, cover and pass on to ascend in a warm spot for around 30 minutes, or multiplied in size.

Thump down mixture on a floured surface, and ply until smooth. Partition into equivalent pieced and shape into balls (the right method is to just barely get chunks of mixture through a circle made by your thumb and index finger, utilizing oiled/buttered hands, this way you get decent smooth chunks of batter). Pack the balls firmly into 2 portion tins of around 22 cm each. Cover and pass on to ascend for around 30-45 minutes.

Prepare in a pre-warmed stove at 180 degrees C for 35-40 minutes. Turn out onto wire racks, and then brush quickly with syrup.

Pass on to cool somewhat, then eat warm, or break into pieces and dry out in a cool stove at 70 degrees C short-term.

33. ROOSTERKOEK

Recipes for Roosterkoek (Bread made on the grill while braying) Roosterkoek for the braai or "Stok Brood" (Pieces of dough pressed onto a stick so that children can braai their own bread)

Ingredients:

- 500g Self-rising flour
- 1 jar of Brew
- 1 teaspoon Salt
- You can add a handful of ground cheddar, spices, honey, molasses, garlic or any of your yummy most loved fixings

Technique:

Add every one of the fixings together and blend well. Place the batter in a dish and cover it with a fabric.

After placing it in a warm oven that has been preheated to a very low temperature, allow it to rise until it is twice as big. It will require around 60 minutes, contingent upon your mixture.

Prepare a flour-sprinkled baking sheet on a flat baking sheet.

Take the baked dough out of the oven.

Try not to ply the mixture.

Sever little pieces without straightening it and put on pre-arranged baking plate. Rehash until all the mixture has been utilized. I truly do sprinkle a little flour on the top as not to dry it out.

The dough should continue to rise in the oven.

Keep in mind, Cook your Roosterkoek moves first before you begin braying.

At the point when the fire is prepared, clean the barbecue.

Cautiously put the little Roosterkoek rolls on the barbecue without contacting it on the top. Turn the Roosterkoek rolls utilizing braai utensils by holding it on the sides to turn, that will forestall you from straightening the Roosterkoek rolls. It requires around 10 minutes, contingent upon the intensity of your fire. Kids love it.

Roosterkoek Mixture Recipe

Ingredients

5 cups bread flour, 1 teaspoon salt, 2 teaspoons sugar, 10 grams (one packet), yeast, 1 cup milk, 50 milliliters of oil, 1 egg, and 2 cups lukewarm water

Add the other ingredients after sifting the flour.

In the middle of the ingredients, thoroughly mix the egg, milk, and water.

Knead it at least once every ten minutes.

Place in warm broiler or spot covered. Knead once more when it has doubled in size.

Roll in flour and flatten slightly.

Cut into squares.

34. "SKILPADJIES"

(Mince bacon and bull liver that is flavored)

This is a customary South African recipe for an exemplary mix of mince, bacon and bull liver that is flavored, enclosed by caul fat and simmered or grilled to cook.

Ingredients

- 4 bits of pork caul fat (around 30cm square)
- 100g minced meat (hamburger, venison or ostrich)
- 50g smoked smudgy bacon, finely hacked
- 500g bull liver, cleaned and finely hacked
- 30g spread 1 little onion, finely hacked
- 1 garlic clove, squashed
- 1/2 tsp. 1/2 teaspoon freshly ground black pepper 1/2 teaspoon freshly grated nutmeg salt
- 1/2 tsp. new marjoram, finely slashed
- 1 tbsp. currants onion sauce, to go with

Strategy

Set the caul fat parts of absorb a bowl of chilled water.

The liver and bacon ought to be cut into peppercorn-sized pieces.

In a bowl combine as one the liver, bacon and your decision of minced meat.

To the meat mixture, add the onion, garlic, black pepper, nutmeg, salt, marjoram, and currants.

Divide the mixture into four equal portions and thoroughly mix to combine. Eliminate the primary piece of caul fat from its chilled water shower and wipe off.

Fold over the edges to form a small sealed parcel and secure the edges with a cocktail stick. Repeat with remaining caulk strips until you have four packs. Place the meat mixture in the center of the drippings.

Sit on a baking plate then move to a broiler pre-warmed to 1800 and heat for an hour (they are far superior whenever cooked on a grill).

Insert a metal skewer into the center of the skilpadjie to check for doneness.

Remove the pencil and gently place it on your lower lip.

In the event that the stick feels hot, the skilpadjie is cooked through. Serve hot, joined by rice, a green plate of mixed greens and onion sauce.

35. POTJIE

Across the board Potjie

Ingredients

- 750g bolo or boneless toss of hamburger
- 1 pig's trotter
- 30ml cooking oil
- 2 onions cut

- 10ml salt
- newly ground dark pepper to taste
- 200g uncooked pearl wheat
- 4 tomatoes, stripped and coarsely slashed
- 250ml dry white wine
- 250ml meat stock
- 2 leeks, cut
- 5 child marrows, cut

Strategy

Cut the bolo or throw into 3D shapes and saw the trotter into segments.

Heat the cooking oil in a "potjie" and brown the meat.

Add the onion and broil until it is clear.

Season with pepper and salt upload the pearl wheat and tomatoes.

Heat the wine and meat stock together in a little container over the fire, then empty the fluid into the "potjie" and cover with the top.

Allow the meat to stew over low coals for 3-4 hours, until it is delicate.

Layer the leeks and child marrows on top and stew for an additional 20 minutes.

36. HAMBURGER CURRY SOUP

Ingredients

- 1 pound cubed hamburger stew meat
- 2 onions, slashed
- 2 tablespoons margarine

- 6 cups hamburger stock
- 2 tablespoons curry powder
- 2 cove leaves
- 2 potatoes cut
- 2 tablespoons refined white vinegar
- 2 teaspoons salt

Planning:

In a huge pan or pot, brown the hamburger 3D squares and onions in spread or margarine.

Add the hamburger stock, curry and narrows leaves. Cook at low intensity for 30 minutes. Add the potatoes, vinegar, and salt. Stew for 45 minutes to 60 minutes, until everything is delicate. Serve hot.

37. BILTONG & PEPPADEW TERRINE

Ingredients

- 3 cups soggy hamburger biltong meagerly cut
- 300 g Peppadew Curds
- 1 cup Peppadews, depleted

Directions

Put a sheet of stick wrap on a level working surface. Place 3 columns of biltong in lines to measure a square shape of 15cm x 25cm, and push down. Spread equitably with cheddar.

Top with a line of Peppadews around 5cm from the base. Place two hands under the grip wrap, and crease over towards the middle.

Return the cling wrap to the surface where you are working. Crease the top over to the middle in something very similar way, keeping the grip wrap in salvageable shape. Fold the bottom cling wrap carefully over and fold the sides in.

Form the terrine in a frankfurter shape with two hands. Refrigerate for the time being.

Just before serving, remove the plastic and slice it with a sharp knife.

38. BILTONG

History and Clues

The word BILTONG is gotten from the words "BIL" (Butt cheek) or meat and 'TONG" or strip.

So it is only a segment of meat. In the United States, also known as "Jerky."

For a really long time humanity has tried to save meat. For centuries, seafarers consumed pickled meat in large wooden caskets during their time at sea. No wonder they experienced scurvy!!

African legends has it that moving African tribesmen, crowding their stock, would put strips of venison under the seats on their ponies as the teasing would soften the meat and the sweat of the creatures would zest it! This should be when veggie lovers were conceived!!

There is nothing similar to genuine South African Biltong and you can make it yourself! BILTONG as we realize this delicacy today is a rich legacy from spearheading South African progenitors who sun dried meat during their journey through the African Subcontinent.

The fundamental flavoring is an emotional mix of vinegar, salt, sugar, coriander and different flavors.

Different salt water recipes and marinades were made and given over for ages!

BILTONG and DROE WORS (dried South African hotdog) is most sought after delights in Southern Africa.

Clues and ways to make BIlTONG

THE MEAT

Biltong can be produced using essentially any hamburger or venison yet recollect, the better the cut and grade of the meat, the better the Biltong!

Silverside is awesome.

Continuously utilize newly cut meat. Please don't utilize vacuum fixed meat. (See "Form" underneath)

Continuously cut the meat with the grain and utilize an exceptionally sharp blade for best outcomes.

Cutting the meat

This is vital. The thicker the meat the more it takes to dry. Go for the gold anything up to 1cm in thickness. Cautious now, as these requirements a touch of fixation. While cutting, one definitely will in general wind up with the lower part of the strip being a lot thicker than the top. Slicing bread is not the same thing! Try to begin cutting meagerly, and to continue cutting till the portion of meat falls away. Try not to hack at the meat, and afterward stop to survey your advancement, and cut further. You will wind up with ugly portions of meat canvassed in scratches and cuts.

Marinating the meat

While marinating the meat generally put the thicker pieces at the lower part of the dish or plate with the more slender pieces at the top. Continuously utilize a cover to fend off any flies for clean purposes.

Hanging the meat

Continuously drape your meat in a dry, "drafty" region, liberated from bugs and flies. On the off chance that flies lay eggs on the meat you will wind up with worms and you can discard your biltong!

Putting away your Biltong

Biltong or smoked food varieties ought to be eaten in something like seven days of planning to keep away from the chance of shape, particularly during wet and blustery periods or on the other hand assuming that you live in moist seaside regions.

To keep biltong over a lengthy period, rather put a few pieces into a plastic sack, suck out however much air as could reasonably be expected through a straw, seal, and freeze for a really long time.

On the off chance that form ought to happen, it very well may be eliminated by clearing it off with a material which has been hosed with vinegar.

Shape

A couple of basic safety measures will forestall the event of this bothering peculiarity. Biltong, particularly the "wettish" type, can be impacted by shape after it has been bought and not consumed inside a couple of days. It can likewise happen while making your own biltong. The accompanying are the most well-known reasons for shape and remember a few hints for how to forestall it:

Form is bound to happen during sweltering and muggy summer periods, particularly at seaside regions. The "Biltong Making Season" was traditionally in the winter. However, you can now make biltong all year round thanks to new techniques like drying cabinets. Simply try not to place your Biltong Producer in moist soggy environmental factors.

Shape is probably going to happen assuming that segments of meat contact each other during the hanging time frame.

Exceptional consideration ought to hence be taken to guarantee that each piece of meat hangs openly.

Keep in mind, assuming that form fires up it quickly spread to the remainder of the group.

Shape is likewise bound to frame on meat that has been vacuum fixed or pre-stuffed and been lying in its own blood for a couple of days on the virus racks in shops. Assuming that you just approach to vacuum or pre-stuffed meat lay out whether the goriness has gone "crude" when you unlock it. On the off chance that it has, been careful, this is a great shape energizer. Before beginning your preparations for making biltong, you will need to thoroughly wipe the meat with a cloth that has been dipped in vinegar and then pat it dry with a kitchen towel. The best is to constantly purchase new meat at the butcher.

Meat should not be hung in a damp outbuilding or damp room that has been closed for months. The fresher the air and the better the ventilation, the less risk there will be of shape pollution.

Many individuals balance their biltong in the kitchen and that checks out. Fare thee well notwithstanding, on the off chance that the kitchen is extremely reduced the steam from the cooking pots, pots and the waste of time can make unsuitably high sticky circumstances.

Keeping your Biltong Producer in a cooled area is very fine. This will stop mold from growing, especially in humid environments.

On the off chance that you distinguish the main indications of shape framing you can save your bunch by acting rapidly. Wipe of all hints of shape with fabric which has been plunged in vinegar. This eliminates the mold spores, allowing you to continue drying the meat by hanging it.

In the event that shape has seriously debased a clump of hanging biltong it won't dry out, regardless of how long it hangs. Give it to the canines. It's anything but a beautiful sight and it will deteriorate the more it hangs!

39. BILTONG PASTA POTJIE RECIPE

Rich, bubbly, impressive, and costly, a biltong potjie is extraordinary dish for an exceptional event.

Ingredients

- 2 onions
- 2 cloves of garlic, squashed or hacked
- 250 gram mushrooms
- 2 twigs of thyme
- 500 gram biltong
- 1 cup frozen corn or 1 can shelled corn
- 500 gram wound or shell noodles, cooked still somewhat firm
- 1 red capsicum
- 250 ml new cream
- 1 cup of ground cheddar (Cheddar or NZ Delectable)
- Sear onion until delicate over medium intensity.
- Add garlic, mushrooms, capsicum and thyme and cook for around 5 minutes.
- Lessen heat.

- Add corn, biltong and cooked noodles, cream and cheddar and intensity slowly through until cheddar begins to liquefy.

40. BILTONG POTJIE RECIPE

(Utilize a Nr 2 estimated Pot which serves 4-6)

Ingredients

- 3 Onions
- 250g Bacon (cleaved up)
- 1Kg Button or Earthy colored Mushrooms
- 2 Cloves Garlic - squashed or finely ground
- 250ml Hot Hamburger Stock
- 750ml Rice - cooked
- 750g Biltong cut
- 100g Parmigiano Reggiano - finely ground (not the powder you purchase in the store please however newly ground from a wedge of wonderful genuine cheddar!)
- Barely any branches of thyme - leaves took out the stalks
- 200g Cheddar
- 25g Spread

Preparing

Construct your fire and permit the coals to become medium hot Preheat your potjie over the coals

Dissolve the margarine in the lower part of the potjie.

Sauté the chopped onions and bacon until they are limp and translucent and the bacon is cooked. Sauté the mushrooms and garlic until they start to turn a light brown and the liquid has evaporated. Add the beef stock and thyme. Layer the cooked rice and sliced biltong until they are all used up. Add half of the Parmigiano-Reggiano cheese and then the cheddar cheese in a single layer on top.

Cover with the top and permit representing 5-10minutes over low intensity coals. Once the cheese has melted, remove the posy from the heat and let stand until flavor develops, about 30 minutes. If the fire is too hot at this point, the rice will start to burn.

Not long prior to serving utilize a huge wooden spoon to delicately mix the potjie so every one of the layers are combined as one and equally dispersed.

Sprinkle over the remainder of the ground Parmigiano-Reggiano cheddar and present with plates of mixed greens and newly prepared pot bread.

41. BILTONG RECIPE

Ingredients

- 2 kg lean simmering meat. (Silverside, Outdoors or such)(London cook)
- 125 gram rock salt (Any coarse salt will do. The coarser the better)
- 25 ml earthy colored sugar.
- 5 ml bicarbonate of pop.
- 2.5 ml coarsely ground dark pepper.
- 12.5 gram coarsely ground coriander seeds.
- 200 ml vinegar blended in with 50ml Worcestershire sauce.
- Warm water, one liter.

Cut meat into portions of around 1cm thick.

Combine as one every single dry fixing. Rub dry flavor blend into the meat.

Layer meat in bowl with the thicker pieces at the base, sprinkling a little vinegar blend over each layer. Leave in cool spot for 24 hours.

Remove the meat, strain the mixture with the vinegar, and add one liter of warm water to the mixture.

Dunk the meat into the vinegar/water blend focus on any salt flavors that actually stick.

Use a paper towel or your hands to squeeze the meat dry.

Stick meat and hang.

42. BOBOTIE

(Pronounced Bo-boo-tee)

South African Bobotie (serves 6-8)

Bunch A

- 1.5 tbsp. ground ginger
- 1.5 tbsp. delicate earthy colored sugar
- 1 tbsp. 1 tablespoon mild curry powder 1 teaspoon turmeric salt, a pinch of black pepper, 50 milliliters of olive oil, five chopped onions, Group B, two thick slices of soaked white bread, one kilogram of lean beef mince, 150 milliliters of raisins, and two tbsp. Mrs Ball's natural product chutney
- 1 tbsp. apricot jam
- 1 tbsp. Balsamic vinegar
- 1 tbsp. Worcester sauce

- 1 tbsp. tomato glue
- Bunch C
- 250 ml low fat milk
- 2 huge eggs
- 4 dried sound leaves (discretionary)

Preparing

Put every one of the elements of gathering A into a pot and sauté in a major pot. Channel the greater part of the water from the bread and blend the bread in with the other fixings in bunch B. Add all of bunch B with bunch A in the pot and bubble for 20 minutes over medium intensity. Mix consistently.

Put in a stove confirmation dish.

Beat milk and egg together and pour over the mince blend. Put inlet leaves on top of the blend.

Prepare in the broiler for roughly 45 minutes in a preheated stove (1800C or 3500F).

Serve with the recipe for yellow rice.

Yellow Rice (Serves 6) 350 grams of basmati rice 50 grams of butter 1 heaping tablespoon caster sugar

1 tsp. ground cinnamon or 1/2 cinnamon stick

6 cardamom units, shelled and seeds squashed

Only less than 1 tsp. ground turmeric

5 tbsp. raisins

Put every one of the fixings in an enormous container with 1 tsp. salt and 500 milliliters of water, then heat to a boil and let the butter melt.

Mix, cover and pass on to stew for 6 minutes. Remove the intensity and leave, actually covered, for 5 minutes.

Cushion up and tip into a warm bowl to serve.

43. BOEREWORS (HISTORY)

Boerewors (rancher's wiener) is essentially as generally South African as Biltong, Koeksisters, Pap (maize porridge) and Vetkoek (fat cake). "Boeries" as it is tenderly known by local people, is staple passage in South Africa. It is healthy, heavenly and sensibly economical. Most importantly, it poses a flavor like nothing else on the remainder of this planet!

History

Boerewors is one more legacy from our spearheading progenitors who used to consolidate minced meat and cubed "spek" (pork as well as hamburger fat) with flavors and additives (vinegar) which were openly accessible from the then Cape State.

During their trip across the hinterland enormous amounts of wors would be made during their outspan (visit) and that which couldn't be eaten would be hung to dry and brought for food as they proceeded with their investigations.

This kind of wors slowly changed over the decades, and the term "Boerewors" became ingrained in our culture.

Up until the mid-1960's, boerewors in South Africa was referred to just as boerewors and by no other name. In order to produce what they considered to be the finest "boeries" available anywhere, thousands of butchers competed with one another. Contest was wild, the purchaser was cheerful! The exceptional taste of boerewors was improved by making acclimations to the amounts of the customary fixings utilized. Some marvelous "boeries" was, nevertheless is, and created with the makers desirously watching the blend of their enchanted elixirs.

The mysterious in the creation of good boerewors lies in the nature of the fixings utilized. The boerewors taste better when the meat is of higher quality.

"Pap en Wors" is rice porridge served with sauce and flame-grilled sausage.

Pap is "mielie" or maize flour based porridge.

"Boerewors" is a hotdog, commonly made with hamburger and pork, grounded meat and cooked on a "braai" or open intensity, outside.

Add 3 cups of "mielie" maize dinner to some virus water until smooth

Add another 3 cups and some salt.

Place the pot on the stove and heat it up until the pap begins to boil.

Add more water if vital.

Decrease intensity and cook gradually for 1 hour blending and adding more water (if vital) each 10 minutes. Present with sauce.

Sauce

Grind an apple finely hack an onion Squash two cloves of garlic finely slash one tomato Fry in olive oil

Add 1 tablespoon of sugar, pureed tomatoes, and 2 tablespoons soya sauce.

Add 1 container of hacked tomatoes

Flavor with salt and pepper

Simmer until the onions are cooked through and a thick sauce forms.

Place pap on a plate, top with a piece of "boerewors," and serve.

44. DROE "WORS" (DRIED WIENER) RECIPE

Any great quality "wors" of the slight assortment can be hung on a mission to dry. This training dates right back to the period of the Incomparable Trip in the mid nineteenth 100 years.

This is the manner by which Droe "wors" (dried wiener) tasted many quite a while back! In a general sense the zest fixings and the technique for arrangement continue as before as the "boerewors" recipe in any case, the meat fixings contrast.

For the Travelers in those days venison, hamburger and sheep was plentifully accessible, yet pigs were not appropriate organization for themselves as well as their migrant way of life.

Thusly, we utilize similar flavors and technique concerning making "boerewors", however the meat type furthermore, amount is somewhat unique.

Customary Recipe

Ingredients

- 3 kg meat or venison (no pork or veal, it goes rank when dried)
- 100 gr meat fat (no pork or "spek")
- 25 ml salt.
- 5 ml ground dark pepper.
- 15 milliliters of ground and singed corriander (see hints and tips).

- 1 ml ground cloves.
- 2 ml nutmeg powder.
- 125 ml earthy colored vinegar.
- 25 ml liquor (discretionary).
- 25 milliliters of marsala
- 200 gr slender (meager) hotdog housings.

Significant NOTE:

Continuously utilize exceptionally lean hamburger. Notwithstanding, even lean hamburger could have a specific measure of fat in it.

Ensure that there is something like 53/4 fat in the blend any other way you will wind up with a very oily dry "wors"!

Strategy

Solid shape all meat.

Combine as one completely and mince coarsely.

Place meat in enormous bowl.

Include vinegar, brandy, and all dry spices.

Combine as one softly with a two dimensional fork. Place in cooler for +/- 2 hours to mix flavors.

Casings should be soaked in water during this time.

Fit housings to hotdog producer and load up with blend.

Don't finished or under-stuff.

This "wors" is more reasonable for drying than it is for cooking. Because of the shortfall of pork and "spek", it isn't quite as delicious as should be expected "boerewors" and many individuals track down the cooked assortment of this recipe altogether too dry for their preferring.

Likewise, hang this "wors" without a doubt longer than different sorts of "wors" as the vast majority lean toward it drier than the rest. When bent, it ought to snap like a twig.

Ingredients for the Traditional Boerewors Recipe:

- 1 kg meat.
- 1 kg of meat.
- 1 kg of slim pork or beef.
- 500 g spek (firm pork overweight from under the covering).
- 25 ml salt.
- 5 ml ground dark pepper.
- 15 ml corriander seared and ground.
- 1 ml ground cloves.
- 2 ml nutmeg powder.
- 125 ml earthy colored vinegar.
- 25 ml liquor (discretionary).
- 25 milliliters of marsala
- Casings for 200 grams of sausage.

Preparation:

Shape all meat and spek.

Combine as one completely and mince coarsely.

Place meat in enormous bowl.

Include vinegar, brandy, and all dry spices.

Combine as one softly with a two dimensional fork.

Place in ice chest for +/- 2 hours to mix flavors.

Casings should be soaked in water during this time.

Fit housings to hotdog producer and load up with blend.

Never over- or under-pack.

Oxtail "Potjie most likely the most delicious "potjie" recipe

45. DRY OXTAIL PIECES WITH PAPER TOWEL

Put prepared flour in a Zip lock sack, then add the Oxtail and shake to cover with flour.

Heat margarine and olive oil and sauté bacon pieces.

Eliminate bacon and earthy colored Oxtail in coming about fat, eliminate and deplete. Chop four of the carrots finely. The leeks and onions should be chopped coarsely. Sauté the finely diced carrots, leeks, and onions until soft. Add Oxtail, bacon, bay leaf, peppercorns, garlic, tomato sauce, red wine, and sherry. Garnish with bouquet garnish.

Bring to a boil slowly, and then simmer for three to four hours.

1 hour prior to serving cut the excess carrots into 1 inch pieces and adds them and mushrooms and cooks gradually.

Only preceding serving, add cream and mix in.

Before adding the cream, combine some cornstarch with it to thicken the sauce.

Method Preheat the oven to 1800 degrees Celsius Heat the butter in a large frying pan adds the shallots, garlic, ginger, and chilli and sauté until the shallots are soft. Remove and set aside. Once the shallots are cool, add them to the beef along with the "atchar," fresh basil, finely sliced salt, and freshly ground black pepper to season. Roll the meat into 10 equal-sized balls. Wrap each ball in a cabbage leaf. Pour the tomatoes into an you can make it outside in a cast iron pot on the braai, or simply make it on the oven in a cast iron pot that has a level surface. No matter what you do, don't invite too many people because it's so good that everyone will want seconds. While doing this dish on the braai, ensure it's not excessively hot yet have coals prepared to add when required.

Ingredients: 1 kilogram of boneless chicken breasts or 12 chicken portions.

- Mushrooms
- 1 Enormous onion
- 1 Parcel of Cook in Sauce mushrooms and wine flavor
- 500 g Glue Rice
- 250 ml Coconut cream or milk
- Olive Oil
- Cheddar - 1 cup ground
- 2 Tomatoes Dark pepper Planning
- Cut the chicken in little lumps
- Cut the mushrooms, onions, red and green peppers.
- Grind the Cheddar
- Cut the two tomatoes

Technique

Heat the pot and add the olive oil. Saute the onions, red and green pepper until gently brilliant brown, add the chicken pieces, earthy colored them gently. Mix in the mushrooms thoroughly. Pour The Cook into the sauce and add water until covered. The pasta rice should be added to this combination, blend well and cover. Save on sluggish intensity for 45 min to 1 hour or until the pasta is cooked.

Remove the intensity. The tomatoes should be placed on top of the cheddar cheese, tomatoes, and cream. Stir in the cream. Grind with dark pepper and spot under the barbecue assuming that you are making it on the oven, or in any case add hot coals on the top for 30 minutes.

Ingredients for a Braai Pie:

- Sandwich type network with edges
- 2 Rolls of Puff Baked good
- 1 Parcel of Spinach
- 1 or 2 Chicken Bosoms (filets) - discretionary
- 1 Bundle Destroyed Bacon
- 1 Onion
- 1 Red Pepper
- 1 Yellow Pepper
- 1 Bundle of mushrooms
- Feta Cheddar
- Mozzarella or potentially Cheddar to taste

Technique:

Roll the first piece of dough out on the grid after it has been defrosted. try not to thaw out for a really long time in the microwave, else the batter goes spongy… your smartest choice is to allow the batter to thaw out leisurely all alone.

Tip: utilize some Splash and Cook on the matrix prior to spreading out the mixture.

Place half of the raw spinach on the dough and fry the onion, bacon, and peppers together. If you're using chicken in the recipe, fry (or braai) it separately.

Tip: Before placing the spinach on the dough, ensure that it is thoroughly dried off. The less water/dampness you have before you start the better.

Cut chicken into pieces and put on spinach Add onion, pepper and bacon combination. Cleave what's more, add the mushrooms

Tip: You could fry the mushrooms in addition to the bacon, onion, and bacon fat. Add various grated cheeses. Add the remaining spinach. The Spinach ought to cover the batter pleasantly; it makes a difference to keep such a large number of juices from leaking through and getting the batter wet.) Put the second roll of batter on top. Seal the mixture (as though you are making pies)

Tip: Egg wash the batter for that extra brilliant earthy colored impact.

Put it high up on the fire and turn continually until brilliant brown… This isn't a steak: rather turn too much than too little :-) That pretty much sums it up: The significant stuff is the puff baked well and spinach, go ahead and analyze.

46. CHICKEN RABBIT CHOW

Depicted as road food with taste, rabbit chows are quintessentially the food darling's

Ingredients

- 1 entire chicken, cut into pieces and solid shapes or 1kg chicken pieces

- 4 cardamon seeds (green)
- 1 enormous onion, diced
- 3 garlic cloves, squashed
- 5 cloves
- 2 tablespoons curry powder (you might pick between gentle or hot)
- 3 cove leaves
- 1 teaspoon new ginger, cruched
- 4 star aniseeds
- 4 tablepoons bean stew chips
- 2 tablespoons cumin
- 2 tablespoons coriander
- 2 tablespoons turmeric
- 2 green chilies, meagerly cut
- 2 medium carrots, stripped and diced
- 2 medium potatoes, cubed
- 2 enormous tomatoes, cleaned and diced
- Salt and pepper to taste

Strategy

Broil garlic, onion, chilies, stew drops, inlet leaves, cardamom seeds, cloves, ginger, aniseed, cumin, coriander, turmeric in olive oil until the onions are delicate. Toss in the chicken and sear for an additional 5 minutes. Add the remaining ingredients and season thoroughly. On low heat, cook for about 60 minutes.

Embellish with new coriander and serve in a D portion of bread or panini.

47. CHICKEN CURRY POTJIE RECIPE

Chicken Curry Potjie (pot) is an extraordinary method for having the option to engage despite everything partake in an incredible dinner by essentially adding every one of the fixings into a tremendous pot over the chimney and passing on to stew.

Ingredients

- 2kg skinless chicken thighs or bosoms
- 3 enormous ground onions
- 5 skinless tomatoes
- 1 enormous tin tomato glue
- 4 stored teaspoons masala
- 3 cove leaves
- 2 pastry spoons squashed garlic
- 1 table spoon coriander
- 1 teaspoon fennel
- 2 enormous sticks cinnamon
- 2 teaspoons salt
- 2 teaspoons sugar
- 1 liter red wine
- 6 Enormous potatoes cut down the middle

Guidelines

Saute your onions and garlic until delicate, then, at that point, add the flavors and let stew for several minutes. Simmer the tomatoes, tomato paste, and some red wine for about 5 minutes.

Add chicken pieces and potatoes with just the right amount of more wine. Put the top on your potjie, stew on a low intensity for around 45 minutes, checking the fluid level consistently, adding more red wine when required. Around 15 minutes before you are prepared to eat add sugar to taste.

Serve on a bed of rice, cooked along with mustard seeds, turmeric and onion pieces for added flavor.

48. CHICKEN PIE

Perfectly crispy on the outside and richly flavored on the inside, this chicken pot pie is a complete meal on its own.

Ingredients

- 1 chicken weighing 1.5kg
- Salt and pepper to taste
- 1 huge onion
- 500ml heated water
- 125ml white wine
- 8 peppercorns
- 1ml ground mace
- 5 allspice berries
- 15ml sago
- 30ml vermicelli
- 30ml margarine
- 1 egg yolk
- Juice of 1 lemon
- 4 cuts ham
- 2 hard-bubbled eggs
- Puff baked good
- 15ml milk

Preparing

To make the Chicken Pie Wash, scorch and cut the bird into pieces

Sprinkle each piece with salt and pepper and spot in weighty pot

Cleave the onion finely also, add it, the boiling water and white wine to the pot

Tie the flavors in cheesecloth and add Stew the chicken delicately until delicate and the meat tumbles off the bones

Add the sago, vermicelli and 15ml [1 Tbsp] margarine blending cautiously to guarantee the sago and vermicelli don't consume

Eliminate the pack containing the flavors along with every one of the enormous chicken bones

Preheat the broiler to 230oC [450oF]

Beat the egg yolk, put 5ml away and blend the rest in with the lemon juice

Add the egg/lemon blend to the chicken and mix gradually until thick and velvety then eliminate from the intensity

Place the chicken in a pie dish with bits of ham and cut hard-bubbled egg in-between and spot the meat with the excess spread

Place an intensity resistant egg cup in the focal point of the pie dish to keep the cake from listing

Cover the chicken [and egg cup] with the puff cake and trimming with segments of the baked good.

The remaining egg yolk and milk should be used to brush the chicken pie's top. Cut a few slits in the pastry to let steam escape, and bake for 30 minutes.

49. "MIELIE MEAL"

Chocolate "Mielie Meal" Pudding Madiba - Despite being in a foreign country, Nelson Mandela was very specific about using South African ingredients. Pete was approached to make a sweet that depicted the New South Africa. In honor of Mandela, he devised this new take on an old favorite by using "mielie meal."

Ingredients:

- 10x entire eggs
- 10x egg yolks
- 500g dull chocolate
- 500g unsalted spread
- 250g castor sugar
- 40g maize dinner
- 30g cake flour
- Touch of salt

Strategy:

Dissolve chocolate and margarine in a twofold evaporator.

Blend eggs, egg yolks and castor sugar until the sugar is nearly broken down be mindful so as not to whisk the combination too quickly or integrate an excess of air.

When the chocolate is dissolved, gradually add the egg combination, mixing delicately and not beating.

Add salt, maize meal, and flour through a sieve, and gently mix until the flour is fully incorporated.

To allow for expansion, fill well-greased Cariole molds three quarters of the way full with the mixture. Heat at 2500C for seven minutes.

Natively constructed Yogurt

Fixings

- 1 L Full cream milk
- 1 tub plain yogurt

Technique

Heat milk in miniature for 2 D mins.

Add tub plain yogurt and race in rapidly.

Cover with grip endlessly fold towel or cover over bowl to keep warm for the time being.

The following can be added the following day: sugar, honey, chopped fruit and nuts, or chopped herbs and chives for savory yoghurt. Etc.

Refrigerate and appreciate.

To proceed with the cycle, keep one tub of the abovementioned and start from the very beginning once more.

Making Malva Pudding:

- 1 cup flour
- 1 tablespoon bicarbonate of pop
- 1 cup sugar
- 1 egg
- 1 tablespoon apricot jam
- 1 tablespoon vinegar
- 1 tablespoon liquefied margarine

- 1 cup milk.

Method:

Spread an ovenproof glass or porcelain compartment. Filter the flour and bi-carb into a bowl and mix in the sugar. Add the other ingredients, excluding those for the sauce, one at a time while thoroughly beating the egg in another bowl. Utilizing a wooden spoon beat the wet fixings into the dry.

Empty hitter into the baking dish, cover with lubed foil, lubed side down, and heat in a 1800C preheated stove for 45 minutes until very much risen and for an additional 5 minutes on the off chance that not cooked enough.

While perhaps not adequately prepared the pudding will not retain the sauce making it tedious inside.

Sauce

While baking is practically finished, heat the elements for the sauce ensuring all the sugar and spread are liquefied. Take the pudding out of the oven when it is done and top it with the sauce.

With some cream, serve hot or at room temperature.

For the paste: D mug balm D cup milk

- 1 cup sugar
- D cup high temp water
- D cup margarine

50. FAST AND SIMPLE "MELKKOS" RECIPE

"Me/kkos" (milk food) is one of those South African legacy dishes that evoke recollections of family meals 'round the kitchen table and the pleasantness of young life.

The recipe for the generally Afrikaans velvety, smooth, "cinnamonny" blend is frequently passed down from a long queue of grandparents and guardians.

We grew up eating our grandma and mom's "me/ksnyse/s" (noodles bubbled in milk) and "me/kkos", the last option of which we took to a greater degree a jumping at the chance to, because of week after week dosages at our life experience school, and underneath we shared our interpretation of the once seven days.

Simple MEIKKOS RECIPE

Ingredients

- 2L full cream milk
- 1 cinnamon stick
- 2 cardamom cases, softly squashed
- 12SmL sugar
- 300mL cake flour
- SmL salt
- 2SmL margarine

Technique:

Consolidate the milk, cinnamon stick, cardamom units and sugar in a medium pot and intensity gradually to edge of boiling over. Mix the flour, salt, and butter into the dry mixture until it resembles breadcrumbs while the milk mixture is heating. Eliminate the cinnamon stick and cardamom cases from the milk combination. Mix the crumbed mixture with a whisk into the boiling milk and simmer for eight minutes. Eliminate from intensity and serve right away.

To assist:

Serve the "melkkos" with a handle of spread and a sprinkle of cinnamon sugar on top. Spoon it up on chilly winter nights while you're nestled into a couch or before a popping fire.

51. SOUSKLUITJIES (DATED DUMPLINGS WITH CINNAMON AND SUGAR)

These Souskluitjies are best when they are newly made despite everything steaming hot, yet they can be warmed the following day and ought to in any case hold their nostalgic enchantment!

Ingredients:

- 1 D Cup Flour
- 1 Teaspoon Baking Powder
- Spot of Salt
- 3/4 Cup Margarine
- 2 Eggs
- 2 Table Spoons Sugar
- Water
- D Teaspoon Salt
- 1 Stick Cinnamon
- Sugar and Cinnamon blended in bowl to sprinkle
- D Cup softened spread

Technique:

Filter the Flour, baking powder and salt together.

With your fingers focus on the margarine into the flour until it has like pieces

Beat the Eggs and sugar until light and fleecy.

Blend the beaten eggs to the flour combination. Try to daintily utilize a spoon and blend.

Bring water, salt, and cinnamon to a boil in a saucepan about S cm deep.

Put a few teaspoons of your dough into the hot water. You can do everything at one time. Cover and simmer for ten minutes on low heat, ensuring that the mixture does not boil over. Simply direct the temperature so it is stewing gradually, without peeping time after time!

Eliminate the dumplings with an opened spoon and orchestrate in a serving dish. Sprinkle liberally with cinnamon sugar (you will require more than you suspect, in light of the fact that the hitter isn't improved) and shower with the margarine.

Serve immediately after allowing the sugar to melt for a few minutes.

52. FISH CAKES

Fish cakes are fillets of fish or other seafood that are chopped or ground, mixed with starchy ingredients, and fried until golden brown. Asian-style fishcakes typically consist of fish with salt, water, starch, and eggs. It may also include a combination of fish paste and surimi.

Ingredients

- 2S0 ml (1 c) cooked fish, cleaned and boned

- 2S0 ml (1 c) bubbled pureed potatoes
- 1S ml (1 T) cleaved parsley
- 1S ml (1 T) ground onion
- 1S ml (1 T) spread or margarine
- 2 eggs
- Salt and pepper Dry breadcrumbs Fat or oil for searing Lemon cuts

Technique

Piece the fish and join with the pureed potatoes, parsley, onion and spread.

Beat one egg, season with salt and pepper and add to the fish blend.

Form into balls that are round and slightly flatten.

Beat the subsequent egg well, roll each fish cake in the beaten egg and afterward cover with breadcrumbs.

Broil the fish cakes in hot fat in a skillet until brilliant brown on the two sides.

Present with cuts of lemon.

53. SNOEK WITH APRICOT JAM

Snoek is tasty with a dash of pleasantness and a gentle flavor like cumin. Attempt it in the stove or braai it outside.

Ingredients:

- 1 tbsp. of chutney, 1/2 cup (60 ml). 1S ml) apricot jams
- 1 tsp. (S ml) ground cumin
- 2 tbsp. (30 ml) lemon juice
- 1 tbsp. (1S ml) sunflower oil

- D tsp. (2.S ml) salt
- Dark pepper to taste

Technique

1, 2 kg entire new snoek or line fish, head eliminated and butterflied

Blend chutney, jam, and cumin, lemon juice, around 50% of the oil and salt and season with pepper. Apply the remaining oil to a braai grid and place the fish, skin side down, on the grid. Apply the jam mixture to the fish. Grill over medium heat, skin side down, for 1 to 20 minutes.

Turnover and brown for a couple of moments or until the fish chips without any problem. Take care not to consume or overcook the fish.

Present with prepared yam and a green plate of mixed greens.

Tip

To prepare in the stove, brush a huge piece of foil with a portion of the oil. Put fish on foil in a stove dish and brush fish as above. Bake for 20 minutes, or until cooked, at 180 OC. The highest point of the fish will brown in the stove.

54. CURRIED FISH (SALTED FISH)

Salted Fish Bone Curry is a Malaysian renowned dish this is extraordinary delicious to consume with rice and the substances are specifically vegetables.

Ingredients

- 1.78 kg Geelbek (Cape salmon) Kabeljou, Kingklip or any dry white fish

- Salt or pepper
- 4 medium-sized onions
- 128 ml (D c) sugar
- 48 ml (3 T) medium curry powder
- 18 ml (1 T) turmeric
- 20 ml (4 t) salt (or to taste)
- 2.8 ml (D t) cayenne pepper (discretionary)
- 780 ml (3 c) vinegar
- 128 ml (D c) water
- 6 squashed lemon leaves

Technique

Clean and filet the fish. Sprinkle gently with salt and pepper. Strip and cut the onions into slight rings.

Blend the sugar, curry powder, turmeric, salt, cayenne pepper, vinegar and water in a huge level lined pot (don't utilize an iron or aluminum pot).

Add the onion rings and lemon leaves and permit cooking for 20 to 30 minutes.

Cautiously place the fish filets in the combination, guaranteeing that they are very much covered, and cook for a further 20 minutes or until done. Treat with the curry sauce every once in a while and turn the filets if essential.

Pack the fish in layers in containers or a veneer dish, covering each layer totally with the hot curry sauce. Allow the remaining sauce to cool before pouring it over. Seal the container and keep it cool.

The fish is prepared to eat following a few days.

Hake can be utilized. Filet, sprinkle with salt and refrigerate for the time being prior to utilizing.

Then, at that point, add Masala and Garam Masala, ginger and garlic and broil yet be mindful so as not to consume these.

Cook the meat, tomato, and paste until brown at a lower temperature.

Add curry leaves, salt and potatoes and cook until delicate, around 20-30mins. Add a touch of water to assist the potatoes with cooking yet not to an extreme.

At the point when done, a portion of a portion of white bread, dig out and load up with curry. Utilize the bread from the inward to clean up the curry sauce. Coriander is a good garnish.

56. GENTLE SHEEP CURRY POTJIE RECIPE

Sheep curry potjie is a genuine number one of mine; especially simple to do in the colder time of year time and at the point when you need to engage enormous groups without going through hours in the kitchen.

Ingredients

- 780g x 2 cubed sheep (you can utilize half meat and half sheep, yet it is more pleasant on the off chance that you utilize just sheep)
- 4-8 yams stripped and cut in enormous pieces
- 1 D teaspoons ground cumin
- 1 D teaspoons ground coriander seed
- 1 teaspoon stew jam
- 2 teaspoons Garam masala
- 1cm ginger stripped and ground
- 6 garlic cloves squashed
- 2 sound leaves
- 1/4 ground turmeric

- 1 tablespoon oil
- 2 onions hacked
- 800g tin stripped tomatoes

Directions on the best way to make it

Liquidize the tin stripped tomatoes in the food processor.

Sear the onions in the oil eliminate the onions.

Utilize a similar pot to dry fry the spices and flavors briefly.

Add the onions and the liquidized tomatoes.

Add the meat bring to bubble.

Cook for 1 hour on the burner with the cover on the pot.

On the off chance that too dries you can add a portion of some water.

Add yams cook for one more hour or till yams are delicate.

The yam thickens the sauce.

Eat and appreciate. The gentle curry freezes well.

57. SHEEP NECK AND CABBAGE "POTJIE"

A "Potjie" is a 3 legged, round lined cast iron pot where you put your fixings in, and it stews joyfully over coals while everybody lounges around it talking ceaselessly and tasting you know what.

It's substantially friendlier than a bar-b-que where the men ordinarily assemble round the fire and the ladies are generally bustling in the kitchen, however don't be mixed up, this is totally a male space furthermore, and the ladies are simply expected to do the side dishes.

Everybody for the most part has his own "secret" fixings and "Potjie" contests are exceptionally well known at fairs. Any enormous cast iron pot with a thick base and a cover ought to do.

Ingredients

- 2 tbsp. cooking oil
- 2 huge onions, cleaved
- 14 sheep neck cleaves
- 28Og bacon, diced
- 16 little potatoes, stripped and quartered
- 1 little cabbage, cut in 8 pieces
- run of 8 oz. water and lemon juice
- run of blended spices
- salt and dark pepper to taste

Technique

Heat the oil in a medium-size "potjie", then, at that point, broil the onions, bacon and sheep cleaves for about D hour, blending every once in a while. Cover with top and pass on to cook for around 48 minutes.

Open the pot, stir, and then add the potatoes, followed by the cabbage. Spices and flavors, in addition to the water and lemon juice, should be added. (Try not to mix yet)

Cover with top and cook for about additional 2 hours gradually over medium coals, check assuming that there's enough water inevitably, and add more if essential.

Mix thoroughly; the bones should let go of the meat.

Present with earthy colored rice and sweet squashed cinnamon pumpkin.

Recipe for Skewed Meat Sosa ties Sosa ties on the BBQ have never tasted better, especially when there are also Boerewors available. These kebabs can contain many sorts of meat (or vegetables) yet sheep Sosa ties appear to continuously taste the best.

Ingredients: 800 grams of boned lamb shoulder or leg, cut into 28mm cubes; two large onions, one sliced into rings and the other finely chopped; 80 milliliters of olive oil or cooking oil; four cloves of peeled and crushed garlic; one tablespoon of curry powder; one teaspoon of turmeric; one tablespoon of brown sugar; four crushed bay leaves; one tablespoon of lemon juice; two lemons, cut into small wedges; 120 milliliters of meat stock; one packet of dried a Heat the spread in a pot and sauté the cleaved onion, garlic and curry powder for a couple of moments.

Add the turmeric, lemon and meat stock, bring to the bubble.

When the marinade comes to the bubble, pour it over the meat.

Permit to cool and place in ice chest short-term.

At the point when prepared to cook stick the meat, apricots, green pepper and onion rings onto the sticks.

Empty the marinade into a pot, add a mass of margarine and salt and pepper to taste, bring to the bubble and serve warm with the Sosa ties and lemon wedges.

You can either cook the Sosa ties for about ten minutes on a very hot grill or braai them over very hot coals, turning them as you go.

Present with the lemon wedges and for side dishes you can make a bowl of feathery white rice, potato salad, heated potato or little coat potatoes and firm bread to absorb the sauce.

NOTE: In the event that you like hot food, add more garlic, a couple of squashed chilies, squashed curry leaves and a sprinkling of peri powder to the marinade.

58. 'KORINGSLAAI' (WHEAT) SALAD RECIPE

This is an extremely outdated recipe from quite a long time back. You can change you fixings to suit your taste. An extremely famous serving of mixed greens for any event.

Ingredients:

- 280ml uncooked Wheat (On the off chance that wheat isn't accessible, utilize brown Basmati Rice)
- 1 Green Pepper, red or yellow can be utilized, cut in little pieces
- 410g tin of Peaches (pretty much the amount) cut in little pieces (I keep the sauce of the peaches passed on in the tin to add it to the sauce.
- 62 milliliters of Sultanas or Raisons Salt for the Wheat Sauce cooking process:

Method Soak the wheat for at least two hours. Rinse, add enough water to cover, and microwave for 10 minutes on high power. Place the wheat in a strainer and wash under cool water. Add the green peppers, sultanas, and peaches to the bowl. Mix all the ingredients for the sauce together and make sure the sugar is dissolved before adding the condensed milk (optional).

Place the dish in the refrigerator covered.

The taste will work on following a day and will save in refrigerator for no less than 4 days.

Ingredients for Baked Stuffed Onions Four medium, skinned onions 30 milliliters Fresh breadcrumbs, salt, and pepper; 80 grams of grate Cheddar cheese; a small amount of milk; a small amount of butter.

28 grams of butter, 28 grams of plain flour, 400 milliliters of milk, 80 grams of grated cheddar cheese, salt, and pepper Method Boil the onions in salted water for 18 to 20 minutes, removing the onions before they become soft. Channel and pass on to cool. Remove the tops the onions, utilizing a sharp, pointed blade, and scoop out the focuses with a teaspoon. Cleave the onion places finely, blend in with the breadcrumbs, preparing and a portion of the cheddar, and saturate with just enough milk if fundamental. Fill the onions with this blend and spot them in a lubed ovenproof dish. Put little handles of spread on top and sprinkle with the leftover ground cheddar. Prepare in the broiler at 200 C (400 F) mark 6 for 20-30 minutes until the onions are cooked and brown.

To make the sauce

Dissolve the margarine in a pot and mix in the flour. Cook for 1-2 minutes. Eliminate from the intensity what's more, bit by bit mix in the milk. Whenever preferred, utilize a portion of the onion alcohol and make up to 400 ml with milk. Bring to the bubble, mixing constantly, until the sauce thickens. Add the cheddar, salt, and pepper, and cook over medium heat until the cheese is soft. Serve the sauce with the onions.

59. CARROT "BREDIE" (STEW)

Carrot Bredie is a customary South African vegetable dish; it's similar to pureed potatoes however with a more round and satisfying flavor.

Ingredients

- 1 onion, cleaved
- 1 Tablespoon oil
- 8 carrots, washed, scratched, and cleaved
- 2 potatoes, washed, scratched, and cleaved
- Spot of salt
- Spot of dark pepper
- 1 cup water

Instructions to make

Measure the oil into a skillet, and intensity over medium intensity.

Add the hacked onion, and cook until the onion is brilliant brown.

Add the vegetables and the flavoring.

Add the water and mix. Heat the mix with the eventual result of bubbling.

Decrease the intensity and put a cover on the pot, yet leave it slightly open, to permit steam to get away.

Let the bredie simmer until the vegetables are soft and the water has evaporated.

Eliminate from intensity and crush.

Serve quickly with a touch of margarine mixed in.

60. CHAKALAKA

Chakalaka is a staple South African dish made from beans, shining veggies, pepper, onions, and tomatoes. It is a honest and highly spiced recipe. Chakalaka is a thick, spicy sauce made with vegetables.

Ingredients

- 1/4 cup canola oil
- 2 Tbsp. 2 tablespoons chopped fresh ginger cleaved new garlic
- 1 Tbsp. cleaved bean stew peppers
- 1 cup cleaved onions
- 2 cups tomatoes, generally cleaved
- 1/2 cup green peppers, generally cleaved
- 1/2 red peppers, generally cleaved
- 3 1/2 Tbsp. masala
- 1 cup ground carrots
- 2 cups vegan prepared beans, in pureed tomatoes
- 2 tsp. Fresh coriander

How to Prepare:

In the oil, fry the onions, chilies, ginger, and garlic. Add the leaf masala or curry powder of your decision. Enhance the tomatoes and heat for 10 minutes.

Cook the carrots and peppers in addition for ten minutes.

Add prepared beans and cook for 8 minutes.

Eliminate from intensity and add coriander. Actually look at preparing. Present with Bread, pap, Boerewors furthermore, pap, Boerewors Rolls, or anything you desire, hot or cold.

61. COPPER PENNY CARROT SALAD RECIPE

Super serving of mixed greens for these special seasons! This customary South African plate of mixed greens can be filled in as a side dish furthermore, keeping in a jar perfect.

Ingredients:

- (Salad)
- 1 kg Carrots
- 3 Onions
- 3 Green Chillies or on the other hand in the event that you lean toward Green Pepper

Strategy: Salad: Ring the carrots.

Bubble carrots 18 minutes (Not excessively delicate) with a touch of salt. (The most recent six minutes you add the onion rings)

Expurgated onions into jewels and chef with the carrots for 6 minutes.

62. DICE GREEN PEPPERS OR CHILIES.

Add carrots, onions and chilies or green peppers in a low bowl. (Recall not to utilize treated steel bowl, as it will make a response due corrosiveness) A glass Container would be great.

Components: (Sauce)

- 280ml water
- 1 parcel of tomato cream soup
- 200 ml Vinegar
- 280 ml Sugar

- 128 ml Oil
- 10 ml Worcester Sauce
- 7 ml Mustard

Technique:

Add every one of the fixings together and bring to bubble for around 8 minutes.

Cover the vegetables with hot sauce.

Refrigerate for no less than one day.

63. CRUSHED DRY MAIZE/CORN KERNELS (ALSO KNOWN AS "SAMP" OR "BEANS")

These are used to make curried samp and beans. samp) and gradually cooked sugar beans. The fragrance that fills a kitchen as it's cooking brings back esteemed cherished, lifelong recollections for the vast majority South Africans.

Ingredients

- 4 cups cooked samp and bean blend
- 18ml sunflower oil
- 1 onion, finely slashed
- 1 green pepper cleaved
- 1 red pepper slashed
- 3 fat garlic cloves slashed
- 1 tsp red bean stew pieces
- 1 tbles curry powder
- Salt to taste

- 1 410gr can hacked tomatoes
- 3 cups finely hacked spinach
- D cup water
- New coriander slashed

Guidelines

Douse the samp and beans for the time being in loads of water.

Channel the samp and bean blend in the wake of dousing for the time being and place in a huge pot covered with clean water and stew gradually until almost delicate. Delicate and all the water have been ingested.

Daintily fry the onion until delicate and clear.

In a small amount of oil, combine the curry powder, rainbow peppers, garlic, and chili flakes.

Add the tomato and stew on medium intensity for approx. 20mins.

Add the water and let it stew again till thick and sassy.

Mix the samp and bean blend and the spinach through the tomato combination and intensity through for approx 8 - 10mins.

Decorate with the slashed coriander. Serve warm with your decision of fundamental dish.

Tip: To save time cook a 800gr pkt of samp and bean blend, which makes 8 cups when cooked what's more, freeze the rest for some other time.

64. HONEY SIMMERED YAMS

This sweet and warm spiced candied yam recipe is a combination of several popular Thanksgiving classics.

Ingredients

- 4 medium yams, stripped and slashed into wedges
- 2 T margarine
- 2 T honey
- Salt and pepper, to taste

Technique

Preheat the broiler to 180 C. Disseminate the crude potato wedges equally in a microwave and ovenproof dish and microwave on high for around 8 minutes, until cooked through (when they can be handily punctured with a blade).

After removing the dish from the microwave, gently toss it with the honey and butter. Cook the potatoes in the broiler for around 10 minutes and afterward barbecue for a further 3 - 8 minutes until they turn a wonderful brilliant variety.

65. POUNDED BEANS RECIPE

Ewa lilo, also known as bean porridge or boiled beans, is a Nigerian delicacy from the Yoruba speaking region.

Ingredients

- 14 ounces green beans
- 1 potato, medium, stripped and cut
- 1 onion, medium, stripped and cut
- 1/2 teaspoon sugar
- 1/3 teaspoon white pepper (to taste)
- 1/2 teaspoon salt (to taste)

- 1/3 teaspoon nutmeg, as trimming, to taste (discretionary) Spread, to taste

Preparing

Wash and tail beans. Kindly note that you could utilize more;

The quantity is irrelevant. On the off chance that you're cooking for multiple individuals, utilize more beans and perhaps 2 potatoes.

Cut the beans transversely into adjusts - - anything from meagerly cut to 1" long.

Continue cutting beans until they are all cut.

Put in a pot, and cut the stripped potato and onion over the beans.

Add around 1/3 cup water, sugar, white pepper and salt. (Indeed, white pepper is awesome here, however dark pepper is fine). Try not to blend: just put top on and bring to bubble then lower intensity and let stew.

Reduce the heat, cover, and allow the mixture to simmer until everything is very soft.

Squash the beans, potato and onion, yet don't attempt to pummel it almost to death - - there ought to be surface.

Typically, there is insufficient liquid remaining. Channel this off - - I utilize a strainer - - or you can reduce it away over high intensity, yet be mindful so as not to consume the veggies.

Add a decent handle of genuine margarine, fork through, and sprinkle with nutmeg to serve. This basic dish can undoubtedly be made ahead and heated up - - the flavor gets to the next level. Act as a vegetable side dish.

66. OLD FASHIONED BEAN SOUP

This classic ham and bean soup recipe is packed with flavor. It's easy to make and can be made on the stove or in a slow cooker.

Put the meat, bacon, and stock into a pot and bring to a boil. Cover and simmer for 1 hour. Heat oil in a pan and fry onions, celery, and carrots for about 10 minutes.

Ingredients

- 2 lbs lamb (like ham) or 2 lbs pork, Cubed (like ham)
- 3 cuts bacon, Hacked
- 2 quarts meat stock
- 2 tablespoons olive oil
- 1 medium onion, finely Hacked
- 2 stems celery, Hacked
- 1 huge carrot, Slashed
- 2 (18 ounce) jars naval force beans
- 3 teaspoons salt
- 1/2 teaspoon pepper

Preparing

Place meat, bacon and stock in a pot and intensity with the end result of bubbling. Cover and stew for 60 minutes.

Heat oil in skillet and sauté onion, celery and carrot for 10 minutes.

Add vegetables to the meat and stew for 20 minutes.

Add salt and pepper and serve.

67. SIAPHAKSKEENTJIES - TRADITIONAI SOUTH AFRICAN (ONION SALAD)

'Slaphakskeentjies' is a standard South African plate of leafy greens recipe that goes with a braai, and is a piece of the South African's life like Rugby that persevered for the long haul.

Ingredients:

- 12 little pickling onions
- 1/2 cup water
- 1/4 cup wine vinegar
- 1/4 cups sugar
- 1 teaspoon Dijon mustard or 1/2 teaspoon mustard powder
- 1/2 teaspoon salt
- 1 egg, whisked

Technique:

Strip the onions, taking consideration to keep them entirety.

Heat up the onions in salted water until recently finished (still somewhat firm). Boiling them for too long will cause them to break apart. Drain.

Blend water, vinegar, sugar, mustard and salt together over heat, until the sugar is broken up and then, at that point, bubble for 8 minutes.

Allow the blend to chill off and whisk eggs into the cooled combination.

Whisk as you slowly bring it to a simmer over low heat. Assuming you heat it too quick, the egg will isolate. At the point when it has thickened, eliminate it from the intensity.

Give the warm dressing a last rush prior to pouring over the bubbled onions.

Let it cool.

Four cooked sweet potatoes, skin-on and cut into thick slices; four cinnamon sticks; 180 grams of brown sugar; four servings; four tablespoons. Spread salt to taste

Strategy

In a weighty lined metal goulash dish layer a portion of the spread, yam cuts, sugar, salt also, cinnamon sticks. Begin again with spread for the following layer and go on with the sweet potato, sugar, salt and cinnamon until done. Put the lid on the pot and cook it for about two hours on low heat on the stove. If needed, the dish can also be baked in a moderate oven and kept in the refrigerator for two days.

68. RECIPE FOR EAST AFRICAN PILAU AND KACHUMBARI

The onion determines the quality of the pilau. This is also the secret to getting the pilaf brown. I recommend using red onions instead of green onions. Kachumbari is a Kenyan onion and tomato salad. This is a very easy salad that can be made in no time with simple ingredients.

Ingredients

- 1/4 cup vegetable oil
- 2 medium red onions, thinly sliced
- Garlic 4 pieces, thinly sliced
- 2 tablespoons fresh ginger, minced, or 2 teaspoons dried ginger
- 1 serrano pepper, seeds eliminated and finely slashed
- 1 pound beef tenderloin, diced
- 1 tablespoon commercially available pilaf seasoning or Recipe
- 2 bay leaves

- 1/4 cup coriander, chopped
- 1/2 teaspoon salt
- 3 Roma tomatoes, diced
- 3 medium potatoes, peeled and quartered
- Basmati or jasmine rice 2 cups beef broth 4 cups

Preparing

Heat 1/4 cup vegetable oil in a large stockpot over medium heat.

Add the sliced onions and fry until the onions start to turn golden brown.

Add the garlic, ginger and serrano and simmer for another minute.

Add the beef cubes, pilau seasoning, bay leaves, coriander, and a pinch of salt.

Cook, stirring occasionally, until the meat is brown and caramelized.

Add the diced tomatoes, cook for 1 minute, and then add the potatoes, rice, and beef broth.

Once it boils, reduce the heat to low, cover and simmer until the rice is cooked and the water has evaporated.

Fluff it up with a spoon and enjoy it with kachumbari

69. KAIMATI (BROILED DUMPLINGS)

Kaimatis get their remarkable flavor from the style with which yeast is applied on wheat flour. This conventional breakfast dish or day nibble is normal among the Swahili and Bajuni people group and was acquired from

Bedouin culture. It serves the entire family.

Ingredients

- 2 cups (280 g) wheat flour, refined
- 2 cups (447 g) water
- ½ tsp. (3 g) vanilla substance, clear
- ½ tsp. (1 g) cardamoms powder
- 1¼ tbsp. (12 g) yeast, dry
- 5 1/8 cups (1000 g) cooking oil
- 4 tbsp. (56 g) sugar

70. MEAT SAMOSA (SAMBUSA YA NYAMA)

Nothing more scrumptious like the Kenyan substantial samosa! For the most part a metropolitan dish, the substantial samosa fills in as a morning meal thing and an entire day nibble. It is appreciated by the whole family.

Ingredients

- ½ kg minced hamburger
- 30 g coriander, new
- 1 stem (356 g) leek, unpeeled, crude
- 1 clove (5 g) garlic, unpeeled, crude
- ¼ tsp. (1 g) bean stew pepper, new, crude
- 3 cups (475 g) wheat coat, polished
- ½ tsp. (2 g) salt, iodized
- 1¼ cups (264 g) water
- 3 cups (572 g) cooking oil

Samosa pocket planning:

- Put 2 ½ cups flour in a bowl and add 1 cup cold water. Blend into a medium delicate batter.

- Turn batter onto a level surface and massage completely until smooth.

- Make a thick lengthy roll, cut into 9 pieces and make the pieces into little balls.

- Carry out the balls, each in turn into wanted thickness.

- Flour the surface, somewhat oil the highest point of each carried out ball and stacks them on top of each other. Go on until every one of the pieces is set.

- Line the edges by punching light holes.

- Carry them out together to one huge round piece.

- Heat a shallow skillet and toast the moved batter for 2 minutes for every side. Assuming that the shallow skillet is as well little, slice the carried out mixture to fit.

71. WEST AFRICA JOLLOF RICE

This is a one-pot rice dish famous in numerous western Africa nations. Despite numerous regional variations and a culturally sensitive debate over the dish's origins between Ghanaians and Nigerians, jolof rice has become the most well-known African dish outside of Africa. It is widely acknowledged as the Louisianan dish jambalaya's forefather. Present with fish, chicken, hamburger, eggs or turkey.

Ingredients

- 2 medium tomatoes, generally slashed (around 5 ounces each) ½ medium Scotch hat pepper (or on the other hand utilize a habanero pepper), stem eliminated ½ medium onion, generally cleaved 3 little red ringer peppers, generally cleaved (around 5 ounces each) ½ cup vegetable oil
- 1 ½ teaspoons salt
- 1 teaspoon curry powder
- 1 ½ teaspoons hot ground bean stew pepper, like African dried bean stew or cayenne
- 1 ½ teaspoons garlic powder
- 1 tablespoon in addition to 1 loading teaspoon onion powder
- 2 straight leaves
- ½ teaspoon ground ginger
- 1 tablespoon dried thyme
- 2 ½ cups medium-grain rice
- Water (depending on the situation)

Preparing

2. Add rice and onions. Blend until the unmistakable shade of rice starts to become white.

3. Add garlic, ginger, and pilau masala. Until the garlic is cooked, continue to stir.

4. In a different bowl, blend the coconut milk with ½ cup of chicken stock.

5. Add the coconut combination to the rice.

6. Turn down the heat in the pot and cover it. Adding chicken stock ½ cup at a time to the rice until it is cooked.

72. PILAU RICE

Tanzania like a lot of Africa, Zanzibar is home to a unpredictably differentiated blanket of culture and food. Pilau rice is a famous hot rice dish informed by the country's rich Indian motivations. Make pilau rice to go with curried meats or with your most loved appetizing vegetable dishes.

Ingredients

- 1/2 teaspoon pilau masala (½ teaspoon cumin seeds, ½ teaspoon entire dark peppercorns, 1 tablespoon entire cloves-in no way related to garlic,
- ¼ teaspoon ground cinnamon, ¼ teaspoon ground cardamom)
- 2 to 3 cups Chicken stock (bubbling) (Vegetable stock for Veggie lover recipe)
- ½ cup Coconut milk (canned)
- Salt
- 1 cup Basmati rice

- 2 tablespoon olive oil
- ¼ cup Onions
- 1 tablespoon Squashed garlic
- 1 tablespoon Squashed new ginger

Preparing

In a huge blending bowl, measure 5 cups of flour.

2. In another bowl, blend salt, 3 tablespoons of oil, and 1 ½ cup of water, mix until the salt breaks up.

3. Pour blend in the flour bowl. Blend well; also, add the excess water until mixture turns out to be delicate.

4. Massage the batter for 10 - 15 minutes; If necessary, add flour.

5. To form a ball, divide the mixture into 11 to 15 equal parts, lay them out on a flat surface, and then cover them with plastic wrap or a clean white cloth.

6. Place the ball on a flat surface that has been lightly floured after removing it. Dust moving pin with flour to keep it structure staying. With a moving pin, roll the mixture more slender than ¼ centimeters (it's OK on the off chance that it's not totally round).

7. Apply oil to the top.

8. As an afterthought confronting you, make one centimeter crease, then continue onward with both two hands.

9. Make four. The remainder will be rolled while cooking.

10. Heat a non-stick skillet on medium intensity (utilize a round flapjack dish). After it is warmed, sprinkle a couple of drops of water on it. The pan is ready if the drops dry quickly.

11. Place the chapati you have quite recently moved on a warmed dish. If the chapati's bottom is golden brown and its top is translucent, flip it over after about a minute.

12. After brushing the top of the chapati with a small amount of oil, check to see if the bottom is cooked and golden brown.

13. In the event that indeed, flip the chapati over once more, presently brush the oil on the second side of the chapati, and turn it over once more.

14. The chapati should be removed from the pan after about 30 seconds and placed on a plate with foil paper over it.

73. CURRY POTATOES

East Africa well-known unleavened seared level bread found in nations like Tanzania, Uganda, Mozambique, Kenya and Burundi. In contrast to the Indian chapati this variety is made with regular flour. Serve with stews, vegetables and meats.

Ingredients

- 5 cups all-purpose flour (non-self-rising), 2 cups warm water, 12 teaspoon salt, and 2 cups canola/vegetable oil (heated and cooled). You won't use all of this.
- 2 cups more flour to use in the kneading.
- 4 tablespoons vegetable oil
- 1 medium onion, hacked
- 1 huge clove garlic, minced

- ½ teaspoon ground turmeric
- 1½ cups of water
- ⅛ teaspoon ground cayenne
- ¼ teaspoon ground cinnamon
- ½ teaspoon ground coriander
- 1 tablespoon tomato glue
- 2 teaspoons lemon juice
- 4 tablespoons new parsley, minced
- Salt to taste

Preparing

Heat oil in enormous skillet over medium intensity.

2. Sauté the onions for 6 to 8 minutes.

3. Add garlic and cook 30 seconds.

4. Add the turmeric, cayenne, cinnamon and coriander and mix well. Add the tomato glue and lemon juice and mix again to join everything.

5. Stir once more before adding the potatoes and about 1/4 teaspoon of salt.

6. Include 112 cups of water.

7. Cover and cook for approximately 10 minutes, or until the potatoes are tender and the pan's juices have thickened and coated them.

8. at the end of the cooking time, stir in the parsley. Serve hot.

Uganda curry potatoes are a famous and simple to make Ugandan side dish. Serve it hot with meat stew or grilled chicken. The heat of this dish an ideal differentiation to a better marinade.

2 lbs. red potatoes, washed, cut into 1 inch blocks, furthermore, parboiled in salted water till nearly, yet entirely not very delicate (Bubble water, add potatoes, cook about 4 minutes, channel, wash with cold water)

Douse the plantain pieces in a bowl of salted water for 15 to 30 minutes.

2. Rinse thoroughly and pat dry.

3. Heat the oil in a sauté dish or skillet over medium intensity.

4. Sauté the plantain slices in batches for 10 to 12 minutes or until cooked through but not browned.

5. Add the plantains, garlic and a tad of olive oil to an enormous mortar or bowl and crush with a pestle or on the other hand potato masher until genuinely smooth. (On the other hand, beat with a food processor.)

6. Add salt and stir in the pork cracklings.

7. Form into 3-inch balls or pile on a plate and serve warm with moistened hands.

74. PUERTO RICO

Puerto Rico is a traditional afro-Puerto Rican dish made with pork chicharrn and fried green plantains. Mofongo works out in a good way for chicken or fish stock, dropped in soups, or served straightforwardly in a mortar.

Ingredients

4 green plantains that have been peeled and sliced diagonally into rounds 3 tablespoons of olive oil 3 to 5 minced cloves of garlic 1 cup of pork cracklings (chicharrones) Salt to taste.

Preparing

Remove the center of the cabbage and hack into pieces-but you lean toward them, put away.

2. Cut onion, put away.

3. Cut carrots, put away.

4. Set aside the peeled and diced potatoes.

5. In an enormous pot heat the oil (medium to high).

6. Add the onions and carrots. For five minutes, sauté.

7. Add flavors (cumin, turmeric, curry) and mix for 1 moment.

8. To prevent things from burning, add water to the pan, which will collect at the bottom.

9. Add potatoes, and cabbage and mix.

10. Add seriously preparing assuming you wish or salt and pepper.

11. Lessen intensity to low-drug, cover with a tight top, and let it cool down for 25 moments or until potatoes furthermore, cabbage is delicate which will really rely on how enormous you cleave potatoes.

12. Allow it to chill down subsequent to taking it the intensity. Salt and pepper can be adjusted according to taste.

A healthy vegan dish that is easy to make, inexpensive, and full of flavor. Produced using

75. ATAKILT WAT ETHIOPIA

Cabbage, carrots, and potato, Atakilt Wat has a flavor profile all its own. Present with other Ethiopian dishes, rice, and injera flatbread!

Ingredients

- 1 head green cabbage
- 1 onion
- 5 potatoes
- 3 carrots
- 1 tablespoon turmeric
- 1 tablespoon curry powder
- 1 teaspoon cumin
- ⅓ cup olive oil
- salt and pepper
- ½ cup water

Preparing

At One with Food: Drench the lentils short-term.

2. Bubble lentils the following morning until delicate: Around 20 minutes.

3. Heat Olive oil and sauté the onion, garlic, jalapeno until clear, around 5 minutes.

4. Add flavors, sauté: 2 minutes.

5. Add the bubbled and depleted lentils and cook for around 10 minutes.

6. Taste and change preparing.

7. Take off oven and let it cool.

8. Include the leaves of the cilantro.

9. A nonstick baking sheet should be prepared and the oven should be at 400 degrees.

10. By dipping your fingers in the dish of water and spreading the water around the perimeter of the spring roll sheet, generously dampen the edge.

11. Place one heaping teaspoon of the filling on the sheet for the spring roll.

12. Close the sheet so that it's presently a triangle. Squeeze the edge firmly and set on the baking sheet.

13. Rehash until you run out of filling.

14. Brush the sambusas generously on all sides with olive oil.

15. Heat until brilliant brown, around 6-10 minutes, then, at that point, flip and brown on the opposite side for pretty much 2-3 minutes.

16. These are extraordinary served warm or at room temperature.

76. LENTIL SAMBUSA ETHIOPIA

Flimsy, flaky batter loaded down with lentils furthermore, Ethiopian flavors. This hand-held canapé, likened to samosas, is a flavorful, mouth-watering tidbit or hors d'oeuvre.

Ingredients

- 1 ½ cups Beluga lentil doused for the time being (Accessible Entire Food sources)
- 1 ½ cups Puy lentils
- 4 finely diced Jalapenos
- 1 onion finely diced

- 3 cloves finely diced Garlic
- 1 cup finely hacked Cilantro
- 1 teaspoon Cardamom Seeds: Ground to a coarse powder 12 teaspoons cinnamon Salt to taste 1 teaspoon black pepper

Preparing

About ten sheets of spring roll oil for frying LENTIL SAMBUSA ETHIOPIA fourteen At One with Food: Pre-absorb the beans warm water (ideally short-term)

2. Strip the beans by placing them into a food processor alongside 2 cups warm water.

3. Run food processor for 3 minutes and check to ensure the greater part of the beans are parted. On the off chance that not, run food processor for several minutes.

4. Add the beans and water to a large bowl and stir with your hand.

5. Pour the water through a sifter, gathering free skins and rehash this cycle until every one of the isolated skins are taken out from the beans.

6. Join beans, red ringer pepper, onion and 1 cup water in a blender, mix until you have an exceptionally smooth combination.

7. Empty the combination into a huge bowl. Break 2 crude eggs into the combination. Put away.

8. In 2 tablespoons of boiling water, dissolve the salt, palm oil, crayfish, and bouillon cube. Allow to cool. Once cooled, add to combination.

9. With a spatula or electric blender, blend the combination completely to integrate air into the combination and cushion the coming about moin for around 10 minutes. Taste and adapt to preparing.

10. Add 4 cups water to an enormous pot, set on high intensity and heat to the point of boiling.

11. Oil a portion skillet, empty portion of the combination into the portion dish, include the cut bubbled eggs. Pour in the remainder of the combination. The loaf pan should be completely covered with aluminum foil.

12. Place the blend filled portion dish in the pot of water (it ought not be shrouded in water), place a tight top over the pot and decrease the intensity to medium. Steam for 45-an hour

13. Eliminate from intensity and put away to cool.

77. MOIN MOI/MOI NIGERIA

Moin is a famous Nigerian steamed bean pudding made from a combination of washed and stripped dark peered toward peas, onions what's more, ground peppers. a protein rich staple frequently served at gatherings, meals and other extraordinary events went with jollof rice, broiled plantains and custard.

Ingredients

- 1 ½ cups dark peered toward beans
- ½ Medium onions (slashed)
- 1 slashed red chime pepper
- 1-2 Scotch hat pepper
- 2 bubbled and de-shelled eggs cut
- 2 Crude eggs
- 1 tablespoon ground crawfish
- 3 tablespoons palm oil
- 3 tablespoons softened spread (discretionary)

- 1 bouillon block (Maggi)
- Salt (to taste)
- 1 cup of water

Preparing

At One with Food: Pick over lentils to eliminate any stones and wash well.

2. Stick cloves into the onion half.

3. Combine lentils, 12 onions, and cloves in a large saucepan.

4. Heat to the point of boiling over medium intensity.

5. Diminish the intensity to low and stew, revealed, until the lentils are delicate, around 20 minutes.

6. Dispose of onion with cloves.

7. Let the lentils cool slightly after draining.

8. In a bowl, consolidate lemon juice, olive oil, mint, cumin, coriander, salt and garlic.

9. Toss in the lentils to combine.

10. Add the roasted peppers and the remaining half of the onion to the lentils by finely chopping it.

11. Chill somewhere around 30 minutes to permit flavors to mix.

12. Serve chilled or at room temperature.

78. LENTIL SALAD MOROCCO

A far off cousin of tabbouleh, this chilly lentil Salad is a sound veggie lover choice stacked with Protein fueled lentils and astonishing flavors. Serve chilled for evening gatherings, potlucks, or appreciate alone.

Ingredients

- 1 ¼ cups green lentils
- 1 little onion, cut fifty
- 3 entire cloves
- 5 cups water
- ¼ cup new lemon juice
- 2 teaspoons olive oil
- 1 teaspoon dried mint
- 1 teaspoon ground cumin
- ½ teaspoon ground coriander
- ½ teaspoon salt
- ½ teaspoon minced garlic
- ½ cup slashed simmered red pepper (about ½ pepper)

Preparing

Whisk together peanut butter and stock and hold.

2. Salt and pepper are used to season the meat.

3. Heat the oil in a huge pan over medium intensity.

4. On all sides, brown the meat thoroughly; try not to swarm the meat; sauté in clusters if essential.

5. Keep warm by removing the meat.

6. Add the onion, peppers, garlic, and carrots to the container and sauté until the onions are clear.

7. Combine the stock and peanut butter.

8. Return the held meat (and any juices) to the pot. Thyme, bay leaf, and the liquid from the tomatoes should be added.

9. Bring to a boil and thoroughly stir. Decrease intensity to low and stew, mixing frequently, for around 1 hour or until the meat is delicate.

10. Taste for preparing.

11. Eliminate the thyme twig and the inlet leaf and dispose of.

12. Serve hot over rice.

79. MAFÉ SENEGAL

A standard lively stew made with a tomato-peanut butter sauce. Stew is made from beef, lamb, or chicken, with many versions facing western Africa. Present with rice or couscous.

Ingredients

- ½ cup peanut butter
- 2 cups stock (your decision, ideally unsalted)
- 2 tablespoons canola oil
- 1 cup hacked onion
- 4 garlic cloves, minced
- 2 lbs. hamburger stew meat, managed and cut into 1 and
- ½ inch 3D squares salt and pepper

- 2 cups tomatoes, stripped and diced (or one 14 and ½ oz. container of diced tomatoes with fluid)
- 1 twig thyme
- 1 inlet leaf
- 1 cup green chime pepper, stripped, cultivated and hacked
- 1 cayenne pepper, cultivated and hacked
- 1 cup carrot, stripped and hacked

Preparing

In a blender, combine the curry powder, onions, scallion, salt, pepper, chilies, ginger, thyme, and a small amount of water. Add more water on the off chance that the fixings don't blend well.

2. Focus on the blend to the shapes of meat, let marinade in the ice chest short-term.

3. Scratch the marinade off the meat and save for some other time.

4. In a frying pan, gently brown the meat and butter.

5. Place the meat in a pan and add the potatoes, carrots and saved marinade then add sufficient water to cover the meat.

6. Bring to a boil, then reduce heat and simmer for one to eleven and a half hours, or until the meat is tender.

80. CURRY GOAT JAMAICA

A well-known party dish, the Jamaican variant of curry goat is commonly less harsh than different varieties. It almost always comes with rice, and fried lettuce is often served with it.

Ingredients

- 2 lb. (counting bones) of goat meat - slice in to shapes (sheep might be utilized as a substitute)
- 2 tablespoon curry powder
- 2 diced onions
- 2 scallions (or spring onions)
- ½ teaspoon sal
- ½ teaspoon pepper
- 2 hot chilies (Scotch hat works perfectly)
- 1 tablespoon new ground ginger
- 6 cloves of minced garlic
- 2 branches of new thyme
- 1 tablespoon margarine
- ½ lb. diced carrots
- ½ lb. diced potato
- ½ Cup water

Preparing

Beans should be washed and soaked in water for three to four hours.

2. Channel the beans and spot them in a huge pot of water.

3. Allow the beans to bubble for around 45mins.

4. Wash the leaves of sorghum.

5. Cut the leaves to a length of three to four inches, toss them in the boiling beans, and let them cook together.

6. To give the waakye its distinctive color, add a teaspoon of baking soda if the sorghum leaves are unavailable.

7. Eliminate the sorghum leaves from the beans after 5mins.

8. Add more water and washed rice to the pot with the beans and beans.

9. Permit the combination to cook for 15-20mins (or until the beans are delicate and the rice is cooked and all fluid has been completely ingested).

10. Be certain that the combination doesn't consume and continue to mix while it cooks.

11. Season with salt.

12. Present with pepper sauce, stew, bubbled egg, or fish, chicken, hamburger and vegetable.

81. WAAKYE GHANA

An exceptionally well known Ghanaian dish remembered to have begun from the northern pieces of Ghana.

Waakye is usually had for breakfast or lunch furthermore, presented with stew, spaghetti, stewed wele, and vegetable serving of mixed greens or seared plantains.

Ingredients

- 2 cups of rice
- 1 cup red beans or dark looked at peas or any sort of beans peas
- 4 dehydrated sorghum greeneries or 1 teaspoon of burning pop
- Salt to taste
- 10 cups of water

Preparing

Drench the sticks for somewhere around 20 minutes completely lowered in water prior to utilizing it to forestall consumes.

2. Heat the stove to 450°F. Gently splash or oil baking sheet or cooking dish to forestall the suya from staying to the container.

3. Mix the onion power, smoked paprika, white pepper, cayenne pepper, hot ground pepper, and bouillon/maggi in a medium bowl. Put blend on a plate, Put away.

4. Strip simmered peanuts, then, at that point, grind in an espresso processor with skin on, until finely squashed. Try not to crush the peanuts into glue. Add the ground peanuts into flavor combination.

5. Wipe the steaks off with a paper towel. Before cooking, you should have a completely dry steak. Cut the steak corner to corner into a medium-thick shape.

6. String the steaks onto the sticks around 4 for every stick. Ensuring that all of the meat slices cover the skewer.

7. Apply the spice mixture to the steak skewer; on each side Line a simmering or baking sheet with foil paper. Place sticks on treat sheet, then, at that point, put on the broiling container or baking sheet.

8. Sprinkle with oil and heat on for around 12-15 minutes.

9. Discretionary - Towards the most recent 3 minutes of baking change from baking to oven setting. To achieve an exterior that is a nice crisp brown.

82. SUYA

Nigeria is a famous sweet shish kebab in West Africa. Generally ready by the Hausa nation of northern Cameroon, Nigeria, Niger, and a few sections of Sudan. Suya is a popular street food in Nigeria and has become a national dish.

Ingredients

- 1 tablespoon garlic powder
- 1 tablespoon onion powder
- 1 tablespoon white pepper
- 2 pounds of sirloin steak
- ¼ cup broiled almonds/peanuts
- ½ - 1 tablespoon cayenne
- 1½ teaspoon smoked paprika
- ½ - 1 tablespoon hot ground pepper or cayenne pepper (discretionary)
- 1 tablespoon chicken Bouillon
- 2 tablespoons of vegetable oil to shower on the meat Salt

Preparing

In an enormous bowl, whisk together everything with the exception of the chicken, making a marinade.

2. Toss the chicken with tongs to coat it in the marinade before serving.

3. Cover with cling wrap and refrigerate for the time being, or possibly three hours.

4. At the point when prepared to cook, preheat your broiler to 350 degrees Fahrenheit.

5. Heat a stove save skillet over medium-high intensity until exceptionally hot.

6. Use utensils to move the chicken bosoms out of the bowl and into the hot skillet, holding the marinade.

7. Let cook until nicely browned, about two to three minutes per side.

8. Empty the held marinade into the skillet and spoon the sauce onto the chicken.

9. Switch off the oven, and use stove gloves to move the skillet to the pre-warmed broiler.

10. Give cook access stove for 15-20 minutes (contingent upon thickness of chicken bosoms), or until cooked through.

83. PERI (OR PIRI) SOUTH AFRICA

A zesty dish famous in South Africa as well as Portugal, Peri (or piri) is the named after a bean stew and the sauce containing it. Serve with various side dishes including rice, zesty potatoes and salad.

Ingredients

Two lemon juices, 1 tablespoon white vinegar, 1/4 cup extra virgin olive oil, roughly chopped yellow onion, 1 teaspoon minced garlic, 1 teaspoon salt, 1 teaspoon ground black pepper, 1 teaspoon cayenne, 1 teaspoon bean stew powder, 1 teaspoon paprika, 1 teaspoon ground oregano, and 2 pounds boneless, skinless chicken bosoms.

Preparing

Preheat the stove to 325 degrees Fahrenheit.

2. Heat 2 tablespoons of the oil in a large casserole made of enameled cast-iron.

3. Season the knifes with salt and pepper.

4. Cook the shanks, two at a time, in the casserole over medium heat for 12 minutes or until browned all over.

5. Move to a plate and crash the goulash.

6. In the casserole, heat the remaining two tablespoons of oil.

7. Add the onion, carrots and garlic and cook over moderate intensity, blending around 5 minutes until delicately caramelized.

8. Add the cumin, coriander, cinnamon, allspice and nutmeg and cook, mixing until softly toasted, about 1 moment.

9. over medium heat, stir in the harissa and tomato paste, and cook for 2 minutes, or until lightly browned.

10. Mix in the wine and bubble until decreased to thick syrup, around 4 minutes.

11. Add the tomatoes and 1 cup of the chicken stock to the goulash. Add salt and pepper to taste and bring to a boil.

12. Place the shanks of lamb in the liquid.

13. Cover firmly and braise in the stove for around 3 hours, treating sporadically, until the meat is practically falling off the bone.

14. Move the knifes to a platter and cover with foil. Leave the stove on.

15. Spread the almonds in a pie dish in an even layer and toast for around 10 minutes, or until brilliant.

16. Strain the sauce into a bowl, pushing on the vegetables; skim any fat.

17. Bring the sauce back to a boil in the casserole over high heat for about 10 minutes, or until it is reduced to 1 cup.

18. Keep warm by adding the lamb and vegetables to the sauce.

19. In a little bowl, blend the mint in with the cilantro and almonds and season daintily with salt and pepper.

20. Soften the spread in a medium pot.

21. Cook the shallot for about 2 minutes over medium heat after adding it.

22. Add the couscous and cook for 2 to 3 minutes or until lightly browned.

23. Bring to a boil the water, the remaining 1 cup of chicken stock, and 14 teaspoon of salt.

24. Eliminate from the intensity and add the currants.

25. Cover and let represent 10 minutes.

26. Mix in half of the herb-almond mixture by adding a forkful to the mixture.

27. Hill the couscous in the focal point of a huge platter.

28. Organize the legs of lamb around the couscous and spoon the sauce on top.

29. Sprinkle with the leftover spice almond combination and serve.

84. MOROCCO BRAISED SHEEP KNIFE

Soften in-your-mouth Moroccan style braised legs of lamb take you directly to northern Africa.

You'll fall in love with the aromatic flavors that are woven into each bite, which are both mildly sweet and certain to be spicy! Serve on basmati rice or couscous.

Ingredients

- ¼ cup extra-virgin olive oil
- 4 substantial legs of lamb (around 1 ¼ pounds each)
- Salt and newly ground pepper
- 1 huge onion, finely hacked
- 2 carrots, finely cleaved
- 2 huge garlic cloves, minced
- 1 teaspoon ground cumin
- ½ teaspoon ground coriander
- ½ teaspoon ground cinnamon
- ¼ teaspoon ground allspice
- ¼ teaspoon newly ground nutmeg
- 2 tablespoons tomato glue
- 1 teaspoon harissa or stew glue
- 1 cup dry red wine
- One 28-ounce can entire stripped tomatoes, depleted what's more, coarsely hacked
- 2 cups chicken stock or canned low-sodium stock
- ¼ cup fragmented almonds, cleaved

- 2 tablespoons finely cleaved mint
- 2 tablespoons cleaved cilantro
- 2 tablespoons unsalted spread
- 1 huge shallot, minced
- One 10-ounce box moment couscous
- 1 cup water
- ¼ cup dried currants

KEY WATT BEEF STEW ETHIOPIA
85. KEY WATT HAMBURGER STEW ETHIOPIA

Key Wat is effortlessly ready in a sluggish cooker (simmering pot). Serve with rice and injera (Ethiopian crepe).

Ingredients

- ½ teaspoon ground cumin
- 1 teaspoon ground fenugreek
- ¼ teaspoon ground nutmeg
- ½ teaspoon dark pepper
- ¼ teaspoon turmeric
- 4 tablespoon hot pepper drops
- 2 tablespoon paprika
- 1 teaspoon ginger powder
- 1 teaspoon onion powder
- ½ teaspoon garlic powder
- ¼ teaspoon ground allspice
- ¾ teaspoon cardamom
- ½ teaspoon ground cloves

- 1 teaspoon ground coriander
- ½ teaspoon ground cinnamon

STEWED HAMBURGER:

- 1 lb. stew hamburger, cut into 1 inch blocks
- 1 teaspoon salt
- ½ teaspoon dark pepper
- 2 tablespoon olive oil, isolated
- 1 little onion, diced
- 2 teaspoon minced garlic
- 1 tablespoon berbere (less on the off chance that you're delicate to zest)
- 2 tablespoon tomato glue
- ½ teaspoon sugar
- 2 cups hamburger stock (or 2 cups water and a meat bullion)

BERBERE Preparing:

Join all fixings. Store in a water/air proof compartment.

STEWED Hamburger:

1. Heat 1 tablespoon olive oil in a huge Dutch stove over medium-high intensity.

2. Season the hamburger with the salt and pepper.

3. Brown the meat in clusters in the Dutch broiler, eliminating to a plate to get its juices.

4 Without cleaning the Dutch broiler, add the excess tablespoon of olive oil.

5. Decrease the intensity to medium-low. Add the onions and cook until brilliant brown, around 15 minutes.

6. Cook for a further minute before adding the garlic.

7. To the onions and garlic, add the sugar, berbere seasoning, and tomato paste.

8. Cook until a thick glue structures, around 3 minutes. Add the hamburger stock and meat and heat it to the point of boiling.

9. Decrease the intensity to medium-low to stew.

10. Beef should be simmered for at least two hours.

11. Eliminate the hamburger from the cooking fluid and shred it by pulling the pieces separated with two forks.

12. Simmer for an additional 15 minutes before adding the beef back to the stock mixture.

Preparing

Combine the salt, onion, scallions, chilies, garlic, five-spice powder, allspice, pepper, thyme, and nutmeg in a food processor; grind to a fine paste.

2. While the food processor is on, add the soy sauce and oil consistently.

3. Empty the marinade into a huge, shallow dish, add the chicken and go to cover. Cover and refrigerate for the present.

4. Before proceeding, bring the chicken up to room temperature.

5. Set up a grill. Barbecue the chicken over a medium-hot fire, turning incidentally, until very much carmelized and cooked through, 35 to 40 minutes.

6. Move the chicken to a platter and serve.

TIP: For a smokier flavor, cover the barbecue while cooking.

86. JAMAICA JERK CHICKEN

Maybe the most well-known component of Caribbean food, jerk is a way of getting ready food local to Jamaica in which the meat is dry-scoured or wet marinated with an exceptionally hot zest combination called Jamaican jerk flavor. Jerk cooking and preparing has followed the Caribbean diaspora all through the world. Present with dark beans, rice and broiled plantains.

Ingredients

- 1 tablespoon allspice berries, coarsely ground
- 1 tablespoon coarsely ground pepper
- 1 teaspoon dried thyme, disintegrated
- 1 teaspoon newly ground nutmeg
- 1 teaspoon salt
- ½ cup soy sauce
- 1 tablespoon vegetable oil
- Two thighs and legs weighing 3 1/2 to 4 pounds each
- 1 medium onion, coarsely cleaved
- 3 medium scallions, cleaved
- 2 Scotch cap chilies, cleaved
- 2 garlic cloves, cleaved
- 1 tablespoon five-zest powder

Preparing

Blend olive oil, garlic cloves, coriander, lemon juice, paprika, ground cumin, salt, cayenne pepper, and saffron together until smooth (go ahead and utilize a food processor for this).

2. Place the fish fillets in the refrigerator to marinate in 12 cups of chermoula.

3. Heat a huge profound skillet over medium intensity and add the carrots, potatoes and the excess chermoula.

4. Mix and cover with a top.

5. Pass on to cook for 25 to 30 min, until the potatoes and the carrots are delicate and cooked. Mix periodically.

6. In the interim, eliminate the tissue from the safeguarded lemon, and finely slash it.

7. Partition the potatoes and carrot combination into 4 equivalent parts and put each piece on a baking sheet. Each piece will make a little home for the fish filets.

8. Put one marinated fish filet on top of every potatoes and carrots home.

9. Top the fish with cleaved chime peppers and safeguarded lemon and finish with cherry tomatoes.

10. Shower some additional olive oil (discretionary) and cover the baking sheet with foil.

11. Depending on the thickness of your fish fillets, place in the oven and bake for 12 to 17 minutes.

12. Serve warm with bread or earthy colored rice.

87. CHERMOULA FISH MOROCCO

In morocco, chermoula is a spice sauce that is generally utilized as a marinade with fish. Serve with couscous, warm bread, roasted cauliflower, or rice.

Ingredients

- 3 tablespoons olive oil
- 4 garlic cloves, finely slashed
- 1 bundle coriander, finely cleaved
- 2 tablespoons lemon juice
- 2 teaspoons paprika
- 1 teaspoons ground cumin
- 1 teaspoon salt
- Squeeze cayenne pepper, or more to taste (discretionary)
- Liberal squeeze saffron (discretionary)
- 4 cod filets or any sort of substantial and flaky white fish filets
- 4 medium measured carrots, stripped and ground
- 2 enormous potatoes, stripped, ground and depleted to eliminate abundance dampness
- 3 ringer peppers, cultivated and cleaved (any tone)
- 1 huge saved lemon
- 1 cup cherry tomatoes
- Preheat stove to (400 F)

Preparing

Basically a day (longer if conceivable) ahead of time, place organic product in a huge container. Pour wine and rum over organic product, so it is totally covered. Fruit should be allowed to soak in the jar.

1. Filter together cinnamon, blended zest, salt, baking powder, and flour.

2. Add breadcrumbs and lime skin, and blend in well.

3. Cream spread and sugar in an exceptionally huge blending bowl. Include browning.

4. Using a large wooden spoon, incorporate the soaked fruit in the cream mixture, adding four cups total.

5. Beat eggs for 10 to 15 minutes or until light and fluffy. Vanilla rose water, and sherry

6. Add egg combination to margarine blend, crease in well.

7. Overlap doused organic product into this blend.

8. Step by step overlap in flour combination.

9. Plaque Test: Verify that the wooden spoon is able to stand upright in the middle of the mixture. In the event that not, adds some more flour until the blend can uphold the spoon.

10. Oil baking container and line with oil paper. Line pans with flour and grease.

11. To ensure that cakes do not become dry, place a pan filled with water in the oven's bottom.

12. Empty blend into tins and prepare for 2 hours in a sluggish stove, 300F.

88. JAMAICA RUM CAKE

A treat cake which contains rum, what's more, customarily served during special seasons.

Ingredients

- 1 lb. 1 pound of ground or chopped raisins prunes, ground or cleaved
- 1 lb. currants, ground or hacked
- 1 teaspoon ground or ground nutmeg
- Red Name Wine (or other red cooking wine)
- Wray and Nephew Over proof Rum (or other white rum)
- 8 ounces spread
- 2 cups sugar
- 3 tablespoon searing
- 1 teaspoon cinnamon
- ½ teaspoon blended flavor for baking
- ½ teaspoon salt
- 3 teaspoon baking powder
- 3 cups baking flour
- 1 cup breadcrumbs
- Finely ground skin of 1 lime (or little lemon)
- 12 eggs
- 2 teaspoon rose water
- ½ cup sherry or blackberry cognac
- 2 teaspoon vanilla

Preparing

Mesh and blend ginger root, pepper, and salt in water.

2. In a bowl, combine the spice mixture with the plantains.

3. Utilizing a profound skillet, heat oil (it should be sufficiently profound to permit plantains to drift) to 350 degrees. Broil plantains, turning once, until brilliant brown on the two sides.)

4. Channel plantains on paper towels and keep in warmed broiler until every one of the plantains are seared.

TIP: Try not to broil them at the same time; they shouldn't contact each other while broiling.

89. KELEWELE

A well-known Ghanaian dish, Ghana Kelewele is made of fried plantains seasoned with spices. It is in many cases filled in as a dish with rice and stew or alone as a veggie lover treat or tidbit.

Ingredients

- 4-6 plantains, ready however not past ready, stripped and cut into reduced down 3D shapes
- 1-2 teaspoon Cayenne pepper or ½ teaspoon of red-pepper
- ½ teaspoon stripped ground new gingerroot
- 1 teaspoon salt
- 2 tablespoons water
- Palm oil or vegetal oil to singe

Preparing

Blend salt, sugar, water, and yeast. Put away for 5 minutes.

2. Add flour and blend.

3. Allow the blend to ascend for roughly 1-2 hours.

4. In a huge, sauce skillet empty vegetable oil into a pot, until it is no less than 3 inches (or around 5 centimeters) high (as well little will bring about compliment balls), and put on low intensity.

5. Put a "drop" of batter into the oil to check that it is hot enough. In the event that it isn't adequately hot, the hitter will remain at the lower part of the pot as opposed to ascending to the top.

6. At the point when the oil is sufficiently hot, utilize a spoon to dish up the hitter, and one more spoon or spatula to drop it in the oil, kind of looking like a ball.

7. Sear for a couple of moments until the base side is brilliant brown.

8. The second side of the ball should be fried for a few more minutes until it is golden brown.

9. Utilize an enormous spoon to remove it from the oil. Put them on napkins immediately to absorb a portion of the overabundance oil.

10. Whenever wanted, you can move the completed item in table sugar or powdered sugar to make it better

90. PUFF-PUFF NIGERIA

A conventional Nigerian delicacy like a pan fried donut. A "should have" tidbit while getting ready nourishment for gatherings that can be filled in as a starter or dessert with any primary course.

Ingredients

- 2 cups warm water
- 2¼ teaspoons dynamic dry yeast (1 bundle)
- 3½ cups flour
- ½ - ¾ cup sugar
- ½ tablespoon salt
- Oil for profound broiling

Preparing

In a huge bowl filter in the flour and baking powder, then, at that point, add the cornmeal, sugar and salt. Speed to blend the fixings.

2. Pour in the vanilla and begin adding the water a little at a time as you whisk everything around. (As it stars to take the state of mixture, you should get your hands in there and begin working. If you discover that the 12 cups of water are insufficient, add a little more. The thought is to work it for 5-7 minutes, until you have a very much shaped batter ball that is firm mixture and marginally tacky. Cover with cling wrap or a tea towel and permit the mixture to rest for about ½ hr.)

3. Dust a work surface with flour and separation the mixture ball into 8 equivalent parts.

4. Utilizing your hands, structure each piece into a stogie shape 4-6 inches long or into a ball around one inch thick. Attempt not to make them excessively thick (they will increment in size as they fry.)

5. Heat the vegetable oil on medium and afterward delicately add the formed batter into the container.

6. Permit to cook for around 2-3 minutes before you flip them over. (Each will probably need between 5 and 6 minutes to cook completely.)

7. Utilize a paper towel to deplete off the overabundance oil after they're cooked.

91. DUMPLINGS JAMAICA

A sweet seared maize solace food a street food that is traditionally eaten on the beach with escovitch fish or other jerk meats.

Ingredients

- 3 tablespoons sugar
- 1 teaspoon baking powder
- 1 teaspoon vanilla
- Around 3 cups of veg oil for searing.
- 1 ½ cups flour
- 3 tablespoons cornmeal
- ½ cup water
- ½ teaspoon salt

Preparing

Before combining the ingredients, bring them to room temperature.

2. Add more flour if necessary to the mixture before mixing it all together. The dough ought to be elastic without being sticky.

3. Roll the mixture on a gently floured board until it is about ¼ inch think.

4. Cut into triangles and sear in hot oil. Sear until the two sides are brilliant brown.

5. Drain the mandazi on newspaper or paper towels after removing it from the oil.

TIP: Mandazi are best served warm.

VARIATIONS:

* Shake some crushed sugar over the hot mandazi.

* Put some white sugar into a pack, add a couple mandazi, and shake the sack to cover the mandazi with sugar.

* Add about a ½ teaspoon of cinnamon, ginger, all-flavor, or cardamom to the mixture or a mix of these flavors to add up to a ½ teaspoon.

* To cut mandazi into the shape of standard donuts, use a circular donut cutter.

* Substitute orange, pineapple, or lemon liquid for the extract.

* Incorporate some coconut shredded into the dough.

* Add ground peanuts or ground almonds to the batter.

* You might substitute 1 teaspoon dry yeast for the 2 teaspoons baking powder. You will need to permit the mandazi to ascend prior to cutting shapes and searing.

Also known as an African doughnut with a sweet flavor that can be altered by adding different ingredients.

92. MANDAZI TANZANIA

Mandazi are commonly made in triangular shapes, and because they do not have frosting or glaze, they are usually not as sweet as doughnuts of the United States style. Mandazi can be eaten with practically any food or plunges or basically as a bite!

Ingredients

- 1 egg, beaten
- ½ cup sugar
- ½ cup milk
- 2 tablespoon. spread, dissolved
- 2 cups white flour
- 2 teaspoon. baking powder

93. DAWADAWA JOLLOF WITH GUINEA FOWL

Ingredients

- 380 g guinea fowl meat
- 500 ml vegetable oil
- 20 g ground ginger
- 10 g bouillon tablet

- 20 g cut onion
- Salt to taste

Arrangement

- Cut guinea fowl into pieces
- Grind ginger and onion
- Season meat with ground vegetables and bouillon tablet what's more, permit to represent 20 minutes

Cooking

- Bubble prepared meat until delicate
- Put oil ablaze and permit to warm
- Aerate the oil by searing onion in it
- Broil guinea fowl pieces in hot oil in segments
- Go incidentally to try not to consume
- When cooked, eliminate meat from oil furthermore, place in a colander to deplete

94. SPAGHETTI (PASTA) JOLLOF GUINEA FOWL

Fixings

- 730 g sweet potato
- 120 g new onion
- 160 g new tomatoes
- 200 ml palm oil
- 50 g fish powder (amani)
- 17 g hot pepper
- 10 g bouillon tablet

- 30 g tomato glue
- 1050 ml water
- Salt to taste

Planning

- Wash and strip sweet potato and cut into blocks
- Grind tomato, onion and hot pepper
- Pound dry fish

Cooking

- Put sweet potato 3D shapes into pan and add water
- Put ablaze to bubble
- Add salt, ground vegetables, tomato glue and fish powder
- Permit to cook until sweet potato is delicate
- Use spoon to pound sweet potato against sauce search for gold consistency
- Add palm oil
- Permit to cook, add cleaved onion and permit to stew
- Serve when cooked

Comments

To upgrade the taste and nourishing substance, non-foul verdant vegetables can be added.

95. TZ (TUO ZAAFI)

Ingredients

- 800 g rice

- 3000 ml water Preparation
- Wash, peel, and cut yam into eatable pieces
- Wash peeled yam (again)
- Add washed yam pieces to salt water (2 tablespoons of salt in 1500 ml of water) and allow standing for three minutes cooking
- Heat oil
- Deep fry yam in bits
- Turn occasionally to cook evenly and to avoid burning
- F Sorghum leaf tail is added to extricate its ruddy earthy colored tone, which makes the food look brilliant and furthermore delicious.

96. WAAKYE (RICE AND BEANS)

Ingredients

- 100 ml vegetable oil
- 120 g onion
- 230 g tomatoes
- 15 g hot pepper
- 200 g water

Sauce for waakye

- Salt to taste
- 20 g fish powder
- 30 g tomato glue
- 13 g ginger
- 10 g bouillon block

Planning

- Cut onion
- Wash and toil tomatoes, hot pepper and ginger
- Pound dry fish

Cooking

- Heat oil and add cut onions to sear
- Add ground vegetables and permit to bubble
- Add tomato glue, mix and permit to stew
- Add fish powder, salt, and a bouillon tablet.
- Mix to equitably blend
- Cover and permit to stew over low intensity to cook further
- Add slashed onions and permit to cook for 2 minutes and take off fire

97. BUBBLED PIGEON PEA

Logical name: Local names for Cajanus cajan are: Adua

Ingredients

- 430 g pigeon peas
- Salt (to taste)
- Hot pepper (to taste)
- Onion (discretionary)
- Ground ginger (discretionary)
- Saltpeter (discretionary)
- 16500 ml water
- 200 g gari (discretionary)

Planning

- Pick unfamiliar materials from the pigeon peas and wash
- Absorb pigeon peas water for the time being to relax and cook quicker (discretionary)

Cooking

- Put water ablaze and add pigeon peas to bubble
- Keep on bubbling, adding water until delicate and cooked
- Add saltpeter to help mellowing and lessen cooking time (discretionary)
- Permit it to bubble until pigeon peas are cooked, add salt (1 teaspoon)
- Serve bubbled pigeon peas with seared oil (100 ml palm oil broiled with 30g cut onion) and gari

98. GROUNDNUT SOUP AT HOME MAIN DISHES (SOUPS AND STEWS)

Ingredients: 300 grams of groundnut paste; 100 grams of onion; 10 grams of hot pepper; 130 grams of tomato; 100 grams of smoked fish; 30 grams of fish powder; 30 grams of ginger; 10 grams of bouillon tablet; 3000 milliliters of water; salt to taste Preparation: Mix groundnut paste with water and mash it; grind tomatoes, hot pepper, ginger, Arachis hypogaea Also known as: Neighborhood names: Sima (Northern District), sikaa (Upper East), siimie, jenii (Upper West)

Ingredients

- 200 g bra leaves
- 300 g groundnut glue
- 130 g crude groundnuts
- 200 g tomato
- 80 g dry okra
- 50 g fish powder
- 60 g dawadawa
- 15 g hot pepper
- 180 g onion
- 10 g bouillon tablet
- Salt (to wash bra leaves and for soup to taste)
- 3500 ml water

Arrangement

- Eliminate terrible fish, fish heads and unfamiliar material or soil from the parcel
- Pound the fish
- Scratch ginger; wash in clean water and drudgery
- Sort crude groundnut
- Sort bra leaves, clean and wash with 30 g of salt water blend also, cut into advantageous pieces
- Pound dawadawa
- Grind hot pepper with tomatoes
- Pound okra (harsh surface)
- Cut onion

Cooking

- Strategy 1: Blend groundnut glue with sufficient water to make a combination of light consistency, stew until oil emerges, blending once in a while

99. FISH BRA LEAVES SOUP

Kenaf

Logical names: Hibiscus cannabinus

Close by names: Bra, bito (Upper East), bri, bre (Upper West)

Technique 2: Add groundnut paste to boiling water and stir to combine; boil until the oil comes out; add ground tomatoes, hot pepper, pounded dawadawa, and fish; add a crushed bouillon tablet; add pounded raw groundnuts, okra, and 1 tablespoon ground ginger (optional); add salt to taste; boil until well cooked; stir in cut kenaf leaves; remove from heat; and serve with tuo zaafi, banku, or rice balls.

Comments

Rather than bra, one can utilize aleefu or any nearby dull green verdant vegetable (not disgusting). Dawadawa is a local condiment made from the seeds of the African locust bean, Parkia biglobosa, which have been fermented. It is generally utilized in country northern Ghana in stew and soup arrangements to work on the taste and fragrance of the food. It is nutritious; sadly, it is being ignored by the metropolitan tip top and step by step by certain individuals in the rustic regions in light of its impactful smell.

Ingredients

- 300 g jute mallow leaves
- 50 g dawadawa

- 150 g new tomato
- 15 g new hot pepper
- 100 g onion
- 50 g fish powder
- 10 g bouillon tablet
- Saltpeter
- 1000 ml water
- Salt to taste

Arrangement

- Wash jute mallow with 30 g salt added to water (saline solution)
- Hack/pound jute mallow
- Grind hot pepper (dry or new) and tomatoes
- Hack onion into pieces
- Pound dawadawa
- Pound dry fish

Cooking

- Put water ablaze to bubble
- Add beat dawadawa and permit to bubble
- Add ground tomatoes and hot pepper
- Add powdered hot pepper and hacked onion and permit to bubble
- In a different pot, steam jute mallow with little water
- Add saltpeter to make it disgusting and steam for around 5-10 minutes
- Add steamed jute mallow to the combination

- Add salt to taste
- Add water (if excessively thick) and permit combination to bubble
- Serve when cooked

Present with tuo zaafi, banku, kenkey or eba

Comments

Meat and additionally any reasonable protein source can be utilized. Palm or some other vegetable oil can likewise be added.

100. FISH JUTE MALLOW LEAVES SOUP (FISH AYOYO SOUP)

Jute Mallow

Logical names: Corchorus olitorius L., C. tridens L., C. trilocularis L.

Normal names: Jute mallow

Nearby names: Ayoyo, Fotsolo, Fontsolo (Upper West)

Ingredients

- 80 g dry okra
- 50 g dawadawa
- 60 g new tomato
- 120 g new onion
- 15 g new hot pepper
- 1 bouillon tablet
- 50 g powdered fish
- Dry onion leaves (gabo)

- 1500 ml of water
- Salt to taste

Planning

- Bubble water
- Cut onions
- Pound dry onion leaves (gabo)
- Pound fish
- Grind tomatoes and hot pepper
- Pound dry okra

Cooking

- Put water ablaze to bubble
- Add beat dawadawa
- Add fish powder and bouillon tablet and permit to bubble
- Add cut onions and ground vegetables
- Add water and permit to bubble
- Add beat dry okra in bits (sprinkling) while at the same time blending to stay away from protuberance development
- Add beat dry onion leaves (gabo) - discretionary
- Permit to bubble for a couple of moments and take off fire

Comments

Gabo (dry onion leaves) is a neighborhood seasoning added to the food to further develop smell and taste.

Fish okra soup (dried) Okra's scientific names are: Abelmoschus callei, A. esculentus

Normal names: Lady's fingers, okra

Local names: Fish okra (fresh) soup 31

Ingredients

- 75 g dehydrated baobab greeneries powder (kuuka)
- 50 g dawadawa
- 50 g fish powder
- 15 g fresh hot pepper
- 120 g fresh onion
- 160 g fresh tomato
- 10 g bouillon tablet
- 100 ml palm oil
- 500 ml water
- Salt to taste Preparation
- Wash and cut okra into pieces
- Smacker okra with saltpetre in a grout or tired

101. COMMON NAMES FOR ADANSONIA DIGITATA:

Neighborhood names: Kuuka (Hausa), tukari (Northern Locale), tukaara (Upper East Locale), tokura zon, tukuru koomo (Upper West Locale)

Ingredients

- 220 g okra
- 200 g garden eggs
- 50 g palm oil

- 130 g new tomato
- 15 g new hot pepper
- 75 g smoked fish
- 30 g fish powder
- 150 g onion
- 10 g bouillon tablet
- 90 g meat (discretionary)
- 10 g ginger
- 500 ml water
- Salt to taste

Planning

- Wash and cut garden eggs and okra into pieces
- Wash fish, eliminate bones and waste, and break into pieces
- Slash onions
- Grind tomatoes, hot pepper, onions and ginger

Cooking

- Put oil ablaze to warm
- Add slashed onions to sear
- Add ground vegetables
- Enhance burnt fish and bouillon dosage and a little water
- Cover and permit to bubble
- Add salt to taste, mix and add cut garden eggs
- Add cut okra and mix when nursery eggs are half-cooked
- Add cleaved onions and permit to cook

- Eliminate from fire and serve

102. PRESENT WITH BANKU, EBA, KENKEY

Fish okra stew

Ingredients

- 550 g amaranth leaves
- 430 g tomatoes
- 200 g onion
- 70 g tomato glue
- 15 g hot pepper
- 50 g fish powder

Planning

- Sort aleefu leaves, clean and wash with 30 g of salt water (brackish water)
- Cut leaves into pieces and whiten
- Wash and toil hot pepper and tomatoes
- Scratch ginger, wash in clean water and toil
- Cut onion
- Grind the agushi into a delicate glue (or dry)

Cooking

- Put palm oil ablaze to warm
- Add onion and permit to broil
- Add ground tomatoes and hot pepper
- Add tomato glue, mix and let it bubble
- Mix, cover and permit to stew

- Add bouillon tablet and salt to taste
- Add agushi, to frame knots and cook without mixing
- Mix to blend equally after knots arrangement
- Add whitened amaranth leaves, mix and permit to stew for a few moments • Bring off fire and serve

Present with plain bubbled rice, bubbled sweet potato, banku or kenkey

Comments

Meat or potentially fish can be filling in for fish powder. All vegetables, especially leafy greens, should be washed thoroughly with enough water, preferably three times; add salt to the last washing water.

103. AMARANTH LEAVES STEW

Amaranth

Logical names: Amaranthus cruentus L., A. lividus, A. dubius

Normal names: Local names for amaranth: Aleefu, aleefi

- 250 g agushi (melon seed)
- 10 g bouillon tablet
- 15 g ginger
- 10 g fresh garlic
- 2700 ml water
- Salt to taste 34 Ingredients
- 300 ml vegetable oil
- 140 g fresh onion
- 250 g fresh tomatoes
- 50 g dry whole hot pepper
- 40 g ginger

- 50 g fish powder
- 10 g bouillon tablet
- 200 ml water
- Salt to taste Prepar

Common names for Adansonia digitata: Tamarind

Nearby names: Preparation

- Scrape and wash ginger
- Wash and grind all spices
- Soak tamarind overnight (optional) Cooking
- Boil water and pour over tamarind
- Soak for several hours (or overnight)
- Mash the mixture to remove the pulp from the seeds
- Add ground spices
- Add more water (3000 ml) and put to boil for 30 minutes
- Remove from fire and allow cooling
- Sieve and strain to remove particles (spices and pulp)
- Sweeten to taste and serve chilled

104. SABDARIFFA HIBISCUS

Common names: Roselle, roan

Neighborhood names: Bra, suure sobolo

Ingredients

- 100 g roselle calyces (dry)
- 40 g new ginger
- 5 g hwentia (African Xylopia aethopica)
- 5 g cloves (colorful Xylopia aethopica)
- 300 g sugar
- 4400 ml water (400 ml used to blend flavors subsequent to crushing)

Planning

- Pick unfamiliar things from the roan leaves
- Wash and scratch ginger
- Grind flavors - ginger, hwentia and cloves

Cooking

- Bubble roselle calyx with ground flavors (technique 1)
- Bubble water and pour over roselle calyces and pass on to represent 45 minutes (or short-term)
- Add ground flavors and mix to blend well (technique 2)
- Cover and pass on to remain until variety is separated
- Pass on blend to cool
- Strain fluid and improve to taste (normal sugars - sugar, honey or natural product juice)
- Add seasoning (discretionary)
- Serve chilled

Various bites presented with porridge.

Left top: flavored sorghum porridge. Upper right: millet porridge with spices. Lower left: flavored corn batter porridge. Right bottom: corn mixture porridge.

SNACKS

105. SIMMERED GROUNDNUTS

Ingredients

- 300 g groundnuts
- 2 tablespoons salt
- 550 ml water
- Ocean/waterway sand

Planning

- Sort new groundnuts and eliminate unfamiliar materials, stones or soil
- Sort to have even sizes
- Sifter and wash sand to clean the sand

Cooking

- Put water (enough) in pot and add salt
- Cover and permit to bubble
- Add groundnuts and permit to bubble for 2 minutes
- Strain water off. Spread out and pass on in the sun to dry
- Heat pot with waterway sand (guarantee the sand is adequately hot)
- Pour in the dried groundnuts and mix (to broil)
- Mix infrequently over low intensity to try not to consume of the groundnuts

- Check for doneness by stripping as well as tasting a seed of groundnut
- Bring off fire when groundnuts are light brown in variety and cooked
- Fill a metal colander or stick bin and shake to separate sand from the simmered groundnuts
- Spread out to cool

Present with corn, millet or sorghum porridge, seared or simmered

106. KOOSE (SEARED COWPEA BEAN CAKE)

Ingredients

- 450 g cowpea (dehusked) flour
- 270 ml oil (for profound broiling)
- 50 g ginger
- 15 g new or dry hot pepper
- 75 g onion (discretionary)
- 1 tablespoon salt
- 1000 ml water

Readiness

- Blend water in with cowpea flour and beat in a round movement until combination is fleecy
- Scratch ginger
- Wash and toil ginger, hot pepper and onion

- Add ground flavors (ginger, hot pepper and onion) and salt to cowpea flour in pieces and keep on beating
- Add water and mix to blend equitably and to get a delicate dropping consistency

Cooking

- Put oil ablaze and aerate by adding hacked onions
- Drop blend by spoonful's in the hot oil and sear, turning periodically until brilliant brown (broiling might take around 3 minutes)
- Take the cakes from hot oil, channel in a colander and put on kitchen paper to remove overabundance oil
- Serve hot with corn, millet or sorghum porridge or alone as a nibble

107. CORN MIXTURE FLOUR PORRIDGE

Ingredients

- 200 g corn batter flour
- 2500 ml water

Readiness

- Blend corn batter in with enough water and sifter

Cooking

- Put water ablaze to bubble
- Add sieved combination to bubbling water furthermore, mix enthusiastically to stay away from development of knots
- Add more water if important

- Mix, and permit to bubble until cooked
- Serve hot

108. PORRIDGE

Flavored corn mixture porridge

Fixings

- 400 g flavored corn mixture
- 2500 ml water

Planning

- Blend corn mixture in with enough water and sifter

Cooking

- Put water ablaze to bubble
- Add sieved blend to bubbling water and mix enthusiastically to stay away from development of knots
- Permit to bubble until it is cooked
- Serve hot

109. FLAVORED SORGHUM BATTER PORRIDGE

Ingredients

- 200 g flavored sorghum batter
- 2300 ml water

Arrangement

- Blend flavored sorghum batter with enough water and sifter

Cooking

- Put water ablaze to bubble
- Add sieved combination to bubbling water and mix overwhelmingly to stay away from arrangement of knots
- Permit it to bubble until it is cooked and serve hot.

110. FLAVORED MILLET FLOUR PORRIDGE

Ingredients

- 200 g flavored millet flour
- 1500 ml water

Arrangement

- Blend flavored millet flour with enough water to shape a mixture
- Pass on mixture to mature (ideally short-term)
- Blend mixture in with enough water and strainer

Cooking

- Put water ablaze to bubble
- Add sieved blend to bubbling water and mix overwhelmingly to keep away from arrangement of knots
- Permit it to bubble until it is cooked and serve hot.

Comments

Porridge is ready in many parts of the country. Spiced porridge is typically referred to as hausa koko in northern Ghana.

www.ingramcontent.com/pod-product-compliance
Lightning Source LLC
Chambersburg PA
CBHW062106220526
45471CB00010B/3617